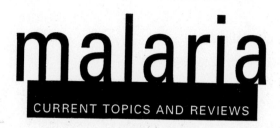

malaria

CURRENT TOPICS AND REVIEWS

Proceedings from
the British Pharmaceutical Conference
September 1996

Edited by
A Louise Sugden and Joseph Chamberlain

PRESS

Published by The Pharmaceutical Press
1 Lambeth High Street, London SE1 7JN

First published 1997

© 1997 The Pharmaceutical Press

Typeset by Techset Composition Ltd, Salisbury

Printed and bound in Great Britain by Page Bros, Norwich

ISBN   0 85369 405 2

Contents

VOLUME 49 ● SUPPLEMENT 2 ● APRIL 1997

J. Pharm. Pharmacol. 1997, 49 (Suppl. 2): 1–2

Introduction to Malaria Symposium

R. D. WAIGH

Department of Pharmaceutical Sciences, University of Strathclyde, 204 George Street, Glasgow G1 1XW, UK

In a history dating back 133 years, the British Pharmaceutical Conference has tended to focus on scientific and technological themes rather than disease states. The 1996 Conference represented a departure from precedent, focusing on malaria, tuberculosis and asthma in separate sessions. The symposia on tuberculosis and asthma are presented elsewhere.

The intention in designing the malaria programme was to provide an overview of the topic by acknowledged specialists as well as more detailed examination of specific issues. The first session, which was given the title "Problems with chemotherapy" (under the chairmanship of R. S. Phillips), began with an overview of drug resistance by D. C. Warhurst.

Chloroquine resistance has been traced to a "multiple drug-resistance" (mdr) gene in *Plasmodium falciparum*, with current work aimed at monitoring drug resistance in field populations. It has recently proved possible to use the polymerase chain reaction to distinguish between resistance arising in old and new infections.

W. M. Watkins gave an account of malaria in local communities in Kenya, from the coast, down to the Rift Valley and as far north as Turkana. The Global Eradication Strategy has been replaced by a policy of Malaria Control, with *P. falciparum* being the major problem, accounting for almost all the morbidity in the region: approximately two million African children die each year from malaria. Quinine remains the standard treatment for severe malaria in East Africa. Chloroquine has been the mainstay of outpatient treatment for 40 years, but resistance is now common, in which case pyrimethamine–sulphadoxine may be used. However, there is an urgent need for alternatives to this combination, with pyronaridine being one possibility.

P. V. Rollason gave the practising pharmacist's view of malaria chemotherapy in southern Africa, particularly in Zimbabwe. There are problems of diagnosis and considerable confusion over the prevalence of drug resistance in this very large geographical area. Unlike Kenya and other parts of the world, the first choice for prophylaxis is pyrimethamine-dapsone.

The first session concluded with an account by D. Walliker of the genetics of *P. falciparum* and the effect on drug resistance of, for example, the sexual phase in the life cycle. Ingestion of blood from patients with more than one genetic form of the parasite will be very likely to result in cross-mating; the ensuing recombination will produce parasites with a wide variety of responses to different drugs. In only a few cases is the mechanism of resistance understood.

The second session, under the chairmanship of D. Walliker, commenced with an overview by a clinician, P. Winstanley, who considered that the situation with malaria would be likely to deteriorate, given economic pressures, global warming and multi-drug resistance. In considering the four strategies of 1) dealing with the vector 2) preventing bites 3) chemoprophy-laxis and 4) symptomatic treatment, he concluded that the latter is the most likely to remain effective in the long term: affordability is the primary requirement.

The status and prospects for malaria vaccines were reviewed by E. M. Riley, who outlined the problems associated with development of a vaccine to an organism which produces surface antigens showing allelic polymorphism and clonal variation in the antigens inserted into the erythrocyte membrane. In addition, the only reliable way to evaluate a candidate vaccine is by a full scale human trial: only one vaccine has undergone multiple field trials, with high resultant specific antibody titres but little or no protective effect.

P. Olliario summarized the newer potential targets for chemotherapy, only a few of which have been fully validated. The approach taken by the World Health Organization Steering Committee on Drugs for Malaria is to combine the efforts of university and government researchers in drug discovery and to develop potential drugs through contracts with industrial partners. A number of high priority targets have been identified, although the absence of an identified target will not be a barrier to development where there is proven efficacy.

The second session concluded with a detailed account of the acute febrile stage experienced by non-immune humans infected with *P. vivax*, presented by R. C. Carter. This febrile stage is probably related to parasite control by the host as an emergency response in the early stages of an infection and coincides with the presence of gametocyte-inactivating mediators in the plasma. The inactivation is dependent on the cytokines interleukin 2 and granulocyte–macrophage-colony stimulating factor, which suggests the possibility of T cell activation.

The third session, under the chairmanship of J. M. Midgley, concentrated on antimalarial drug design directed at a variety of targets. R. G. Ridley began by describing the identification of three proteases involved in haemoglobin degradation: several compounds appear to mediate their antimalarial activity through inhibition of two of these proteases. He went on to describe the remarkable bisquinolines, which bind to free haem, prevent its polymerization, and do not show cross resistance with chloroquine.

Continuing the haem theme, G. Edwards discussed the effect of haemin on the degradation of artemether in-vitro; haemin also potentiates the neurotoxicity of three artemisin analogues in-vitro, as measured by the effect on neurite production in two neurally-derived cell lines, probably by catalysing breakdown of the peroxide bridge.

G. H. Posner then described some elegant studies on the Fe(II) catalysed breakdown of artemisinin, leading to a detailed understanding of the mechanism of formation of, among other species, a potent alkylating epoxide. An understanding of the mechanism has allowed the design of a number of simple, symmetrical endoperoxides with substantial in-vitro antimalarial activity.

The activity of iron chelators as antimalarials both in-vivo and in-vitro led R. C. Hider to consider the design of orally active compounds based on 3-hydroxypyridin-4-ones. Such compounds are relatively non-toxic, but for high efficacy require to be targeted towards the parasite and to fail to gain access to sensitive tissues such as brain and bone marrow. While there is evidence that such selectivity is achievable, the available animal models may be inadequate; parasite biochemistry in rodents may be different from that in primates, with regard to iron transport.

Moving away from the involvement of iron, P. K. Rathod outlined several years work on the synthesis of antimalarials directed at thymidylate synthase. While direct selective inhibition is difficult, it is possible to take advantage of the requirement by the parasite for exogenous orotic acid. As a result, 5-fluoro orotate inhibits *P. falciparum* in-vitro with IC50 of 6 nM and with no distinction between chloroquine-sensitive and -resistant cells. A combination of 5-fluoro orotate and uridine increases selectivity and cures malaria in mice.

B. Kilbey was indisposed and could not present his paper on the malaria replisome as a drug target; the text is included here as a potential guide for antimalarial drug design. DNA synthesis occurs at five stages in the complex life cycle and work continues on cloning and characterizing the genes which encode the replication proteins, followed by attempts at gene expression. These studies are helping to gain information on the patterns of expression in the erythrocyte and the mechanisms which control the expression.

J. Pharm. Pharmacol. 1997, 49 (Suppl. 2): 3–7

Drug-resistant Malaria: Laboratory and Field Investigations*

D. C. WARHURST

London School of Hygiene and Tropical Medicine, Keppel St., London WC1E 7HT, UK

About 40% of the world's population is exposed to malaria, and there are up to 500 million clinical cases per year with 1·5–2 million deaths. The most lethal and well established species in man, *Plasmodium falciparum*, has its main focus in Africa where high mortality is seen in children (World Health Organization 1996).

Transmission depends on the bite of female anopheline mosquitoes and the pre-erythrocytic stage which develops from the sporozoite in the insect's saliva, grows for more than 5 days in the liver without pathological effects. Following escape from the liver, the infective merozoites enter red blood cells and begin a 48-h (tertian) or 72-h (quartan) division cycle: blood schizogony. Fever is seen when the mature dividing stages burst out of the red cells to reinfect others. Red cells containing *P. falciparum* maturing blood stages adhere to capillary endothelium in deep tissues including the brain to avoid capture by the spleen, and cause severe pathology.

Malaria parasites of man originated in the higher primates in the old world. Human genetic data indicate that malaria was carried to the Americas by colonisers (Cavalli-Sforza et al 1994). *P. vivax*, the benign tertian malaria parasite, probably originated from a parasite similar to *P. schwetzi* found in the chimpanzee and gorilla in Africa. In South America, *P. vivax* passed from man to the black howler monkey as *P. simium*, accounting for very close genetic similarities between *P. vivax* and *P. simium* and observations of cross infection to man (Goldman et al 1993). A similar occurrence took place with *P. malariae* which in Africa infects both man and chimpanzee (Garnham 1966). It passed from man into the South American squirrel and other monkeys as *P. brasilianum*, which is very similar genetically. *P. falciparum* apparently separated from the chimpanzee and gorilla parasite *P. reichenowi* in Africa at about the same time that ancestors of chimpanzees and man diverged (Escalante et al 1995). It is restricted to the hominoids and did not infect local monkeys when introduced into South America.

P. falciparum resistance to quinine was first reported in 1910 in persons returning from South America, but refractory strains were later recognized in Europe (Peters 1987). Use of this cinchona-derived alkaloid as a prophylactic was moreover associated with development of blackwater fever, a severe haemolytic crisis during a fulminating malaria attack. New, safe synthetic drugs, chloroquine and the antifolates pyrimethamine and proguanil were introduced after 1945, but only chloroquine appeared free from the problem of resistance. Chloroquine became a standby for prevention and treatment of malaria, and, together with DDT, the basis of a worldwide programme for malaria eradication. Hopes were dashed in the early 1960s when chloroquine-resistance was reported in *P.*

falciparum from highly endemic regions of Venezuela and Colombia in South America and the Thailand–Cambodia border in South East Asia, while DDT began to show failures in several areas. Subsequently, chloroquine resistance spread throughout South America, and to the remainder of South East and South Asia, finally reaching East Africa in 1978 and spreading across to West Africa by 1985 (Payne 1987).

Chloroquine remains usable and is used as a first-line drug in many areas of Africa. In our 1993 study in Zaria, Northern Nigeria, only 7 treatment breakthroughs were noted when 43 children were treated with a standard course (Adagu et al 1995a). However, quinine, once discarded as too toxic (Findlay 1951), is an essential second-line drug, especially in severe and complicated disease. Potentiating antifolate combinations of pyrimethamine with the sulphonamide sulphadoxine have served well in less severe disease and are an invaluable follow-up to quinine, with tetracycline as an alternative. Amodiaquine and other chloroquine analogues are also undoubtedly still valuable for treatment, especially where resistance to chloroquine is not too marked.

There is no doubt that in many areas, quinine is the clinician's first choice for treatment of severe disease. Moreover in Thailand, where quinine replaced chloroquine in 1978, there is now a significant amount of quinine (and, in some cases mefloquine) resistance in border areas with Myanmar and Cambodia (Fontanet et al 1993).

Drug treatment of active cases can assist in the control of transmission in areas of low malaria endemicity. Mosquito control measures, and means of avoiding man-mosquito contact by bednets may be the most effective measures in zones of higher endemicity, where chemotherapy serves for reduction of morbidity and mortality, and drug prophylaxis may be targeted to pregnant women and (in some cases) to small children.

Mechanisms of Drug Action and Resistance

Blood schizontocides

These agents (which include chloroquine, amodiaquine, quinine, mefloquine and halofantrine) act only on the growing intra-erythrocytic stages carrying out haemoglobin digestion. Their effect is rapid, and since the blood stages are responsible for malaria pathology, they are preferred for treatment of severe disease. Although liver stages are unaffected, chloroquine has been used widely as a prophylactic of low toxicity, preventing the development of a clinical infection. This is termed suppressive prophylaxis.

Allison & Young (1964) localized quinine fluorescence in mammalian digestive vesicles—lysosomes according to the definition of De Duve & Wattiaux (1966). Our group (Warhurst & Hockley 1967; Warhurst & Williamson 1970) and Macomber et al (1967) were able to show ultrastructurally that

---

*Dedicated to the late Dr James Williamson, biochemical parasitologist and friend.

the pigment clumping following chloroquine-treatment of rodent *P. berghei* and the simian parasites *P. cynomolgi* and *P. knowlesi* represented fusion of adjacent plasmodial digestive vesicles into an autophagic vacuole, and that rRNA was degraded during the 1- to 2-h process of clumping. We suggested a trapping mechanism for lysosomotropic concentration of weakly basic drugs, involving the accumulation of protonated membrane-impermeable drug within the acidic lysosome contents (Homewood et al 1972). This idea was later expanded by De Duve et al (1974). The incrimination of the lysosome was subject to a vigorous but unsuccessful criticism from Hahn et al (1966), who supported a direct action on DNA. The lysosomotropic hypothesis did not, however, serve as a full explanation of chloroquine's selective activity on malaria parasites (Warhurst 1985), because mammalian cells also have acidic lysosomes.

We compared the ability of blood schizontocidal antimalarials to inhibit chloroquine-induced pigment clumping competitively, and outlined a hypothetical receptor associated with the lysosome (Warhurst & Thomas 1975).

Clues as to the possible nature of the lysosomal receptor had been revealed as early as 1964 in studies on the interaction of chloroquine and quinine with haemin (ferriprotoporphyrin IX), although it was then felt that such an interaction might form a mechanism of resistance rather than a mode of action (Cohen et al 1964). Haemin, a toxic iron porphyrin, is produced within the lysosome during digestion of haemoglobin and is complexed as a non-toxic crystal, malaria pigment or haemozoin (Slater et al 1991). Suggestions that haemin might be a target were first made in 1967, but it was not until 1980 that Fitch and his group (Chou et al 1980) found fairly conclusive evidence, suggesting that drug-haemin complexation prevented haemin from detoxication as haemozoin (McChesney & Fitch 1984). The haemin molecule answered some of the requirements for the lysosomally located receptor we had proposed (Warhurst & Thomas 1975), and it was possible spectrophotometrically to demonstrate its complexation with quinine, other cinchona alkaloids and mefloquine. The absence of interaction with antiplasmodially inactive 9-*epi* quinine was compelling evidence. A ring-ring interaction between quinine and haemin in the organic or membrane phase was proposed and modelled, with coordination proposed between the side-chain nitrogen of the drug and the Fe^{3+} of haemin (Warhurst 1981). The ring-ring interaction has been confirmed subsequently, but the iron coordination apparently involves the adjacent alcoholic -OH group (Constantinidis & Satterlee 1988a). It has also been shown that chloroquine has a similar ring/ring interaction with haemin or haemin dimer in aqueous solution (Moreau et al 1985; Constantinidis & Satterlee 1988b).

Assuming the importance of the haemin interaction, which has been disputed (Warhurst 1986), the probable explanation for the antiplasmodial inactivity of the 9-*epi* cinchona alkaloids relates to the short distance between the 9-OH (9-hydroxyl group) and the side-chain quinuclidine -N, allowing an intramolecular hydrogen bond to form (Oleksyn 1982), which effectively prevents the -OH group's coordination with Fe^{3+}. The similarity in crystallographic parameters of quinine, cinchonidine, quinidine, cinchonine and the related drug mefloquine (Karle & Karle 1991), and the mutual similarity of their calculated minimum energy conformations in-vacuo, and that of halofantrine (Warhurst, unpublished data) allow a

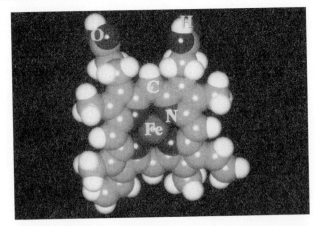

FIG. 1. Ferriprotoporphyrin IX (haemin) structure computed using semi-empirical ZINDO single point calculation.

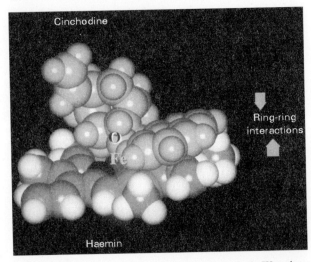

FIG. 2. Cinchonidine structure computed using semi-empirical AMI single point calculation followed by molecular mechanics MM+ geometry optimization.

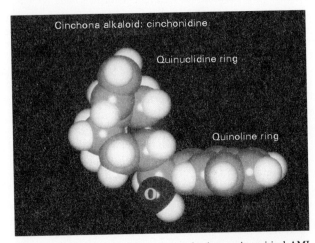

FIG. 3. Docking of cinchonidine with ferriprotoporphyrin IX to show coordination linkage of cinchonidine hydroxyl oxygen with Fe^{3+} of the iron porphyrin.

common model to be suggested where a planar aromatic surface bears a hydroxyl oxygen able to coordinate with the Fe^{3+} in the centre of the haemin ring (see Figs 1, 2 and 3).

A striking feature which makes haemin unlike any other drug receptor is its relative bilateral symmetry which will allow efficient binding of enantiomers. This agrees with observations on antimalarial activity, since ($-$) (natural) and ($+$) (unnatural) quinine are equipotent (Warhurst 1987). It is fascinating to note that the apparently crucial interaction between the sesquiterpene endoperoxide qinghaosu antiplasmodials such as artemisinin with haemin also depends on an iron-oxygen reaction (Posner et al 1994; Shukla et al 1995). It is also relevant that, even though they are not basic, the artemisinin derivatives are effectively concentrated by malaria-infected erythrocytes (Gu et al 1984).

Resistance to blood schizontocides

Blood schizontocides can be divided on chemical grounds into the following groups: 4-aminopyridine analogues (chloroquine, amodiaquine, amopyroquine, mepacrine); and aryl amino alcohols (quinine, mefloquine, halofantrine). Infections moderately resistant to 4-aminopyridine analogues are treatable using aryl amino alcohols.

Chloroquine-resistant malaria parasites take up less chloroquine (Fitch 1970; Diribe & Warhurst 1985) than do sensitive ones. This may be due to enhanced export of the drug from the cell, mediated by an MDR protein (multiple drug resistance or P-glycoprotein) as is found in some drug-resistant cancer cells. This was suggested when verapamil, known to reverse drug resistance in cancer cells by interfering with the activity of the MDR protein, was found to reverse chloroquine-resistance in-vitro in *P. falciparum* malaria (Martin et al 1987). Chloroquine-resistant parasitized erythrocytes were observed to release chloroquine at least 40 times as fast as sensitive ones (Krogstad et al 1987), but there is disagreement about this. A characteristic *mdr* gene has been detected on chromosome 5 in all *P. falciparum* strains examined. Mutations in Pfmdr1 have been linked to chloroquine resistance (Foote et al 1990) in some areas (Adagu et al 1995b, 1996; Basco et al 1995) but not in others (Awad El Kariem et al 1992; Wilson et al 1993). It appears that another gene may permit chloroquine resistance, and mutations in Pfmdr1 may be secondary, since an area of chromosome 7 contains a site linked in a laboratory cross to chloroquine resistance (Wellems et al 1991). In addition, amplification of Pfmdr1 is in some cases associated with resistance to mefloquine, halofantrine and probably quinine (Wilson et al 1993).

Antimetabolites

Antimetabolites attack all growing stages of the malaria parasite. They will even inhibit the early growing stages in the liver (causal prophylactic effect) and the developing infective stages in the mosquito (antisporogonic effect). The type I antifolate sulphonamides inhibit dihydropteroate synthase (DHPS). The type II antifolates, pyrimethamine and the proguanil metabolite cycloguanil, inhibit a later enzyme, dihydrofolate reductase (DHFR) (the pathway from para-amino benzoic acid (PABA) to the tetrahydrofolate co-factors is essential in the synthesis of the pyrimidine deoxythymidylate for DNA). The similarity of antiplasmodial sulphadoxine/pyrimethamine (SDX/PYR) combinations to the poten-

tiating antibacterial type I + II antifolate package cotrimoxazole is clear.

Resistance to antimetabolites

Resistance to these drugs apparently depends largely on point mutations in the DHPS and DHFR genes (Peterson et al 1990; Brooks et al 1994). Combinations of type I and type II antifolates have been generally effective against pyrimethamine resistance, and at first resistance to SDX/PYR was not a significant problem (Kilimali & Mkufya 1985). Now it seems, particularly in East Africa and South East Asia, that resistance to SDX/PYR is becoming more widespread. Is this due to higher levels of resistance to the PYR component, reflected in additional mutations in DHFR, or is it due to development of resistance to SDX as well?

Resistance Monitoring Using Techniques Based on Molecular Biology

We are interested in developing molecular biological techniques to monitor drug resistance to currently-used antimalarials in field populations using easily applicable low-technology blood-spot sampling methods (Warhurst et al 1991) and polymerase chain reaction (PCR)-based genetic analysis protocols carried out in central laboratories. The aim is to make resistance monitoring and consequent modification of treatment guidelines more efficient.

Since resistance changes are often linked to point mutations in specific genes, methods for PCR detection need to be mutation-specific. Currently we employ PCR followed by restriction digests to detect mutant and wild-type alleles (Frean et al 1992) but we are also testing a colorimetric ELISA-based system (Aguirre et al 1995) modified using mutation-specific primers.

In addition to examining resistance-related mutations, we can use PCR to look at the antigenic diversity of the malaria parasites to detect whether drug breakthroughs are due to development of resistance in existing parasite clones in the blood, or to new infections. This technique (Babiker et al 1995) combined with resistance-mutation detection, has proved to be most illuminating. In our recent Gambian study it confirms that chloroquine failures which occur 28 days after initiation of treatment, are mostly new infections (Duraisingh et al unpublished).

References

Adagu, I. S., Warhurst, D. C., Ogala, W. N., Abu-Aguye, I., Audu, L. I., Bamgbola, F. O., Ovigwho, U. B. (1995a) Antimalarial drug response of *Plasmodium falciparum* from Zaria, Nigeria. Trans. R. Soc. Trop. Med. Hyg. 89: 422–425

Adagu, I. S., Warhurst, D. C., Carucci, D. J., Duraisingh, M. T. (1995b) Pfmdr1 mutations and chloroquine resistance in *Plasmodium falciparum* isolates from Zaria, Nigeria. Trans. R. Soc. Trop. Med. Hyg. 89: 132

Adagu, I. S., Dias, F., Pinheiro, L., Rombo, L., do Rosario, V., Warhurst, D. C. (1996) Guinea-Bissau: association of chloroquine-resistance of *Plasmodium falciparum* with the Tyr86 allele of the multiple drug resistance gene Pfmdr1. Trans. R. Soc. Trop. Med. Hyg. 90: 90–91

Aguirre, A., Warhurst, D. C., Guhl, F., Frame, I. A. (1995) Polymerase chain reaction-solution hybridization enzyme-linked immunoassay (PCR-SHELA) for the differential diagnosis of pathogenic and non-pathogenic *Entamoeba histolytica*. Trans. R. Soc. Trop. Med. Hyg. 89: 187–188

Allison, A. C., Young, M. R. (1964) Uptake of dyes and drugs by living cells in culture. Life Sciences 3: 1407–1414

Awad El Kariem, F. M., Miles, M. A., Warhurst, D. C. (1992) Chloroquine-resistant *Plasmodium falciparum* isolates from the Sudan lack two mutations in the pfmdr1 gene thought to be associated with chloroquine resistance. Trans. R. Soc. Trop. Med. Hyg. 86: 587–589

Babiker, H. et al (1995) Genetic evidence that R1 chloroquine-resistance of *Plasmodium falciparum* is caused by recrudescence of resistant parasites. Trans. R. Soc. Trop. Med. Hyg. 88: 328–331

Basco, L. K., le Bras, J., Rhoades, Z., Wilson, C. M. (1995) Analysis of Pfmdr1 and drug susceptibility in fresh isolates of *Plasmodium falciparum* from Sub Saharan Africa. Mol. Biochem. Parasitol. 74: 157–166

Brooks, D. R., Wang, P., Read, M., Watkins, W. M., Sims, P. F., Hyde, J. E. (1994) Sequence variation of the hydroxymethyldihydropterin pyrophosphokinase: dihydropteroate synthase gene in lines of the human malaria parasite, *Plasmodium falciparum*, with differing resistance to sulfadoxine. Eur. J. Biochem. 224: 397–405

Cavalli-Sforza, L. L., Menozzi, P., Piazza, A. (1994) Development in South America. In: The History and Geography of Human genes. Princeton University Press, Princeton, New Jersey, pp 313–316

Chou, A. C., Chevli, R., Fitch, C. D. (1980) Ferriprotoporphyrin IX fulfils the criteria for identification as the chloroquine receptor of malaria parasites. Biochemistry 19: 1543–1549

Cohen, S. N., Phifer, K. O., Yielding, K. L. (1964) Complex formation between chloroquine and ferrihaemic acid in vitro, and its effect on the antimalarial action of chloroquine. Nature 202: 805–806

Constantinidis, I., Satterlee, J. D. (1988a) UV-visible and carbon nmr-studies of quinine binding to urohemin-I chloride and uroporphyrin-I in aqueous-solution. J. Am. Chem. Soc. 110: 927–932

Constantinidis, I., Satterlee, J. D. (1988b) UV-visible and carbon nmr-studies of chloroquine binding to urohemin-I chloride and uropor-phyrin-I in aqueous-solutions. J. Am. Chem. Soc. 110: 4391–4395

De Duve, C., Wattiaux, R. (1966) Functions of lysosomes. Annu. Rev. Physiol. 28: 435–492

De Duve, C., De Barsy, T., Poole, B., Trouet, A., Tulkens, P., Van Hoof, F. (1974) Lysosomotropic agents. Biochem. Pharmacol. 23: 2495–2431

Diribe, C. O., Warhurst, D. C. (1985) A study of the uptake of chloroquine in malaria infected erythrocytes. High and low affinity uptake and the influence of glucose and its analogues. Biochem. Pharmacol. 34: 3019–3027

Escalante, A. A., Barrio, E., Ayala, F. J. (1995) Evolutionary origin of human and primate malarias: evidence from the circumsporozoite protein gene. Mol. Biol. Evolution 12: 616–626

Findlay, G. M. (1951) Recent Advances in Chemotherapy. Vol. II, Churchill, London

Fitch, C. D. (1970) *Plasmodium falciparum* in owl monkeys. Drug-resistance and chloroquine-binding capacity. Science 169: 289–290

Fontanet, A. L., Johnston, D., B., Walker, A. M., Rooney, W., Thimasum, K., Sturchler, D., Macdonald, M., Hours, M., Wirth, D. F. (1993) High prevalence of mefloquine-resistant falciparum malaria in Eastern Thailand. Bull. WHO 71: 377–383

Foote, S. J., Kyle, D. E., Martin, R. K., Oduola, A. M., Forsyth, K., Kemp, D. J., Cowman, A. F. (1990) Several alleles of the multidrug-resistance gene are closely linked to chloroquine-resistance in *Plasmodium falciparum*. Nature 345: 255–258

Frean, J. A., Awad El Kariem, F. M., Warhurst, D. C., Miles, M. A. (1992) Rapid detection of Pfmdr1 mutations in chloroquine-resistant *Plasmodium falciparum* malaria by polymerase chain reaction analysis of blood spots. Trans. R. Soc. Trop. Med. Hyg. 86: 29–30

Garnham, P. C. C. (1966) Malaria Parasites and other Haemosporidia. Blackwell, Oxford

Goldman, I. F., Qari, S. H., Millet, P. G., Collins, W. E., Lal, A. A. (1993) Circumsporozoite protein gene of *Plasmodium simium*, a *Plasmodium vivax*-like monkey malaria parasite. Mol. Biochem. Parasitol. 57: 177–180

Gu, H. M., Warhurst, D. C., Peters, W. (1984) Uptake of [^{3}H]dihy-droartemisinine by erythrocytes infected with *Plasmodium falciparum* in vitro. Trans. R. Soc. Trop. Med. Hyg. 78: 265–270

Hahn, F. E., O'Brien, R. L., Ciak, J., Allison, J. L., Olenick, J. G. (1966) Studies on the modes of action of chloroquine, quinacrine and quinine and on chloroquine-resistance. Milit. Med. 131 (Suppl.): 1071–1089

Homewood, C. A., Warhurst, D. C., Peters, W., Baggaley, V. C. (1972) Lysosomes, pH and the antimalarial action of chloroquine. Nature 235: 50–52

Karle, J. M., Karle, I. L. (1991) Crystal structure and molecular structure of mefloquine methane sulfate monohydrate: implications for a malaria receptor. Antimicrob. Agents Chemother. 35: 2238–2245

Kilimali, V. A. E. B., Mkufya, A. R. (1985) In vivo assessment of the sensitivity of *Plasmodium falciparum* to sulfadoxine/pyrimethamine combination (Fansidar) in six localities in Tanzania where chloroquine-resistant *P. falciparum* has been detected. Trans. R. Soc. Trop. Med. Hyg. 59: 482–483

Krogstad, D. J., Gluzman, I. Y., Kyle, D. E., Oduola, A. M., Matin, S. K., Milhous, W. K., Schlesinger, P. H. (1987) Efflux of chloroquine from *Plasmodium falciparum*: mechanism of chloroquine resistance. Science 238: 1283–1285

Macomber, P. B., et al (1967) Morphological effects of chloroquine on *Plasmodium berghei* in mice. Nature 214: 937–939

Martin, S. K., Oduola, A. M., Milhous, W. K. (1987) Reversal of chloroquine-resistance in *Plasmodium falciparum* by verapamil. Science 235: 899–901

McChesney, E. W., Fitch, C. D. (1984) 4-Aminoquinolines. In: Peters, W., Richards, W. H. G. (eds) Antimalarial Drugs II. Springer, Berlin, pp 3–60

Moreau, S., Perly, B., Chachaty, C., Deleuze, C. (1985) A nuclear magnetic resonance study of the interactions of antimalarial drugs with porphyrins. Biochim. Biophys. Acta 840: 107–116

Oleksyn, B. J. (1982) The role of molecular geometry in the biological activity of cinchona alkaloids and related compounds. In: Griffin, J. F., Duax, W. L. (eds) Molecular Structure and Biological Activity. Elsevier, Amsterdam, pp 181–190

Payne, D. (1987) Spread of chloroquine-resistance in *Plasmodium falciparum*. Parasitol. Today 336: 1451–1452

Peters, W. (1987) Chemotherapy and Drug Resistance in Malaria. Academic Press, London

Peterson, D. S., Milhous, W. K., Wellems, T. E. (1990) Molecular basis of differential resistance to cycloguanil and pyrimethamine in *Plasmodium falciparum* malaria. Proc. Natl Acad. Sci. USA 87: 3018–3022

Posner, G. H., Oh, C. H., Wang, D., Gerena, L., Milhous, W. K., Meshnick, S. R., Asawamahasadka, W. (1994) Mechanism-based design, synthesis, and in vitro antimalarial testing of new 4-methy-lated trioxanes structurally related to artemisinin: the importance of a carbon-centered radical for antimalarial activity. J. Med. Chem. 37: 1256–1258

Shukla, K. L., Gund, T. M., Meshnick, S. R. (1995) Molecular modeling studies of the artemisinin (qinghaosu)-hemin interaction: docking between the antimalarial agent and its putative receptor. J. Mol. Graph. 13: 215–222

Slater, A. F. G., Swiggard, W. J., Orton, B. R., Flitter, W. D., Goldberg, D. E., Cerami, A., Henderson, G. B. (1991) An iron-carboxylate bond links the heme units of malaria pigment. Proc. Natl Acad. Sci. USA 88: 325–329

Warhurst, D. C. (1981) The quinine-haemin interaction and its rela-tionship to antimalarial activity. Biochem. Pharmacol. 30: 3323–3327

Warhurst, D. C. (1985) Drug resistance. Pharm. J. 235: 689–692

Warhurst, D. C. (1986) Antimalarial schizontocides: why a permease is necessary. Parasitol. Today 2: 331–333

Warhurst, D. C. (1987) Cinchona alkaloids and malaria. Acta Leiden-sia 55: 53–64

Warhurst, D. C., Hockley, D. J. (1967) The mode of action of chloroquine on *Plasmodium berghei* and *P. cynomolgi*. Nature 214: 935–645

Warhurst, D. C., Thomas, S. C. (1975) Pharmacology of the malaria parasite. Biochem. Pharmacol. 24: 2047–2056

Warhurst, D. C., Williamson, J. (1970) Ribonucleic acid from *Plasmodium knowlesi* before and after chloroquine treatment. Chem. Biol. Interact. 2: 89–106

Warhurst, D. C., Awad El Kariem, F. M., Miles, M. A. (1991) Simplified preparation of malarial blood samples for polymerase chain reaction. Lancet 337: 303–304

Wellems, T. E., Walker-Jonah, A., Panton, L. J. (1991) Genetic mapping of the chloroquine-resistance locus on *Plasmodium falciparum* chromosome 7. Proc. Natl Acad. Sci. USA 88: 3382–3386

WHO (1996) World Malaria Situation in 1993. Weekly Epidemiological Record Parts I, II, III & IV. WHO, Geneva, pp 3–5 and 17–48

Wilson, C. M., Volkman, S. K., Thaitong, S., Martin, R. K., Kyle, D. E., Milhous, W. K., Wirth, D. F.l (1993) Amplification of Pfmdr1 associated with mefloquine and halofantrine resistance in *Plasmodium falciparum* from Thailand. Mol. Biochem. Parasitol. 57: 151–160

J. Pharm. Pharmacol. 1997, 49 (Suppl. 2): 9–12

Malaria in East Africa

W. M. WATKINS*† AND K. MARSH*‡

*Clinical Research Centre, Kenya Medical Research Institute, Nairobi, Kenya, †Department of
Pharmacology & Therapeutics, University of Liverpool, UK, and ‡Nuffield Department of Clinical Medicine,
University of Oxford, UK

Historically, malaria has coloured the European view of East Africa since the days of early exploration. Victorian England regarded the African coast as a place where they were very likely to die from the disease, and with good reason. The protestant missionary, Rev. Dr Johann Ludwig Krapf, arriving in East Africa in early May 1844 before the rains started, established a mission station at Rabai, outside Mombasa. He was "attacked by the fever" on 1st July, and his pregnant wife became sick at the same time. She gave birth to a baby girl on 6th July, but died 3 days later. The baby died on 15th July. It was felt that no European could live long on the coast of East Africa without being attacked by *mkunguru* or fever of the country (Pavitt 1989).

Obviously, the major burden of malaria morbidity and mortality falls on the people of Africa; a disease which still kills approximately two million African children each year, despite the considerable resources which are directed against it. The Global Eradication Strategy for malaria, conceived as a practicable endeavour, has quietly been replaced by a policy of Malaria Control. Vector control has been largely abandoned as impracticable, drug resistance in the parasite continues to erode the small collection of effective treatment drugs and a malaria vaccine remains well below the horizon. Despite hopeful new initiatives (bed nets, improved drug availability to rural areas), malaria remains a scourge for the inhabitants of East Africa.

Malaria Epidemiology in East Africa

The pattern of malaria within the region varies considerably. All of the four species of *Plasmodium* which cause disease in man are found in East Africa: *P. falciparum*, *P. malaria*, *P. ovale*, and *P. vivax*. *P. vivax* is rare and found only in individuals whose red cells carry the Duffy factor, but does occur in coastal regions, where Arabic genetic influence is strongest. *P. falciparum* is the most important infection by far, and is responsible for most of the malaria morbidity, and virtually all the malaria mortality of the region.

In Kenya, there are areas of "stable" malaria, where the climate supports mosquito proliferation, and there is year-round transmission: the lake Victoria basin; the coast; and narrow strips of land along the major rivers. Over the rest of the country, malaria is often found where there is surface water (e.g. after the annual rains) and where the altitude is low enough to support an adequate mosquito population. In these areas, malaria tends to be "unstable". It is often highly seasonal, as is the case in Turkana, Northern Kenya, a semi-desert region where parasite rates are very low during the 10 months

Correspondence: W. M. Watkins, Clinical Research Centre, Kenya Medical Research Institute, Nairobi, Kenya.

of the year when no rain falls. Epidemic malaria may arise in these areas. This is a particularly dangerous occurrence because the people have little immune protection and mortality can be high.

The relationship between the malarial parasite, the human host and transmission by anopheline mosquitoes is well-established. Less well understood are the specific interactions between the host and the parasite, a major focus of research. Young children are the age group most often parasitized. Typically, parasite prevalence by age increases sharply as protective maternal immunity wanes (ca. 6 months), reaching a peak before the age of 5 and then declining. The peak itself is a function of the transmission characteristics of the area. In Kilifi, Kenya coast, (year-round transmission but with pronounced seasonality), this occurs later than in Ifakara, Tanzania which has year-round, high transmission. In Kilifi, the average young child has one or two clinical attacks of malaria each year, although there will be parasitaemic episodes which do not give rise to sickness. These asymptomatic parasitaemias become more common after childhood with increasing exposure to the local parasite strains. The outcome is a partial immunity against subsequent attacks, and few children over the age of five die from malaria. There is, therefore, a distinct difference between the parasitized but well child, and the parasitized sick child. By adulthood, while clinical malaria may still occur, it is rarely life-threatening, except in the pregnant woman, where lowered immunity leads to increased parasite densities and sometimes severe anaemia.

A very large number of African children die each year from malaria (estimates vary, but the number is of the order of 2 million deaths; 5617 each day, 234 each hour, 4 every minute). Most of these deaths are caused by *P. falciparum*. To address this major health problem, we need to know more about the factors which are responsible for the progression: uninfected, infected (well), infected (sick), very sick, death. We do not yet know whether the control of this progression is mainly due to host or parasite factors. This is a major research effort of the KEMRI-Wellcome Trust Research Programme, at Kilifi, a research unit on the Kenyan coast.

Clinical Malaria

Malaria is an illness occurring with parasitaemia (malaria parasites seen on microscopic observation of a finger-prick blood sample), which is often serious enough to make the child's mother seek health care. The diagnosis is not straightforward because in endemic areas many children will be parasitaemic, but well, or parasitaemic but sick due to a different condition (e.g. respiratory infection, or measles). At the health centre or hospital, cases are divided, on the basis of clinical presentation, into non-severe or severe malaria. Clinically, the sick child with non-severe malaria usually has fever and general malaise, but without any of the attributes of severe malaria (high parasitaemia, anaemia, metabolic acidosis, seizures and sometimes cerebral complications, including coma). Non-severe malaria is generally managed by a treatment course of an effective antimalarial drug alone. However, because of the time-dependent kinetics of parasite sequestration, there is always the possibility of a non-severe case becoming severe over a short time period. A smaller proportion of malaria patients present to hospital with more serious, life-threatening disease, who require admission; this is 'severe malaria' by definition. In Kenya, life-threatening malaria can be subdivided into three overlapping clinical syndromes; malaria with impaired conciousness, malaria with severe respiratory distress, and malaria with severe anaemia. There is a complex interaction between these components, and the risk of death is proportional to the degree of overlap (Marsh et al 1995). Similarly, cerebral malaria, one of the most serious clinical manifestations, is no longer regarded as a homogenous clinical syndrome. Even strictly defined cerebral malaria, with unarousable coma, comprises several distinct syndromes: 'metabolic' coma, associated with severe metabolic acidosis; coma due to atypical status epilepticus; and a primary neurological syndrome (English et al 1996). Recovery from severe malaria may be complete in terms of easily recognizable defects. However, it is becoming clear that many children suffer from neurological sequelae which may have far-reaching implications for the mental development of the child and the acquisition of educational norms at school.

In other parts of the world, e.g. South East Asia, where falciparum malaria is of lower endemicity, and patchy, individuals are more likely to remain immunologically naive into later life, and adult malaria patients are much more common than in Africa. There is a remarkable difference in the clinical pattern of severe malaria between these two groups. In adults, acute renal failure and acute pulmonary oedema are frequent causes of death (WHO 1990) whereas children more often die of severe anaemia and metabolic acidosis although it is often difficult to ascribe an exact cause of death (White & Ho 1992). The pace of the disease is quicker in children than in adults; the child tends to deteriorate more rapidly, and also recover more quickly than the adult (Waller et al 1995). Another striking difference between these age groups is the rarity of neurological sequelae in adults who recover from cerebral malaria.

Parasitaemia and disease severity
The correlation between clinical severity and parasitaemia is weak in malaria; well children may have high peripheral parasitaemia, and occasional cases of cerebral malaria may be slide-negative. One of the problems in judging the relationship between peripheral parasitaemia and clinical condition is that the blood slide only provides information on the number of circulating (non-sequestered) parasites, and not on the total parasite load. As the parasite matures through the erythrocytic cycle, which is complete in 48 h for falciparum malaria, a stage is reached where parasites express adhesin proteins on the red blood cell (RBC) surface, which stick to specific binding sites on venule endothelium. The net effect is the removal from circulation of RBCs containing the more mature parasite stages. For this reason, patients with the same level of peripheral parasitaemia may differ by 62-fold in their sequestered parasite biomass (White & Krishna 1989). Postmortem specimens from patients who have died from severe malaria may show venules in the brain which are packed with adherent parasitized erythrocytes (PRBCs). In-vivo, it is likely that PRBCs are loosely attached, and roll along the inner vessel wall in the direction of blood flow. The sequestration mechanism is advantageous to the parasite, since it effectively protects it from reticuloendothelial clearance. However, it follows that the peripheral parasitaemia is not a reliable measure of total (circulating plus sequestered) parasite load. This fact creates a problem in using parasitaemia per se as an indicator of disease severity. Although there are methods for estimating sequestered parasitaemia (White & Krishna 1989), none are yet appropriate to bed-side use.

The Treatment of Clinical Malaria

Treatment strategies differ for severe and non-severe malaria, which is the main reason for the two categories.

The treatment of severe falciparum malaria
The accepted rule for the chemotherapy of severe falciparum malaria is to start treatment with an effective drug, immediately the diagnosis is proved or suspected. The parenteral route should be used whenever possible because the absorption of drugs by the gastrointestinal route cannot be relied upon in severely ill patients who may be vomiting, or shocked, and in whom the blood flow to the gut may be reduced (Warrell 1993). The use of a loading dose to rapidly achieve inhibitory blood concentrations has been a contentious issue for quinine in the past, but is still the recommended method (Warrell 1993; Marsh et al 1995). Recent research in Kilifi has shown that the intramuscular route may be unreliable under certain conditions. Absorption of water-soluble drugs from intramuscular depot injections is altered by malaria infection (Winstanley et al 1992), and absorption of drugs having low water solubility from this site may be dangerously reduced in severe malaria because of reduced blood flow to skeletal muscle (Murphy & Watkins, unpublished data). An interesting possibility is the use of the rectal route to deliver drugs in severe cases, where the patient may be unconscious. The methodology is undemanding, and could be used by rural dispensaries (which lack the skills and equipment for intravenous administration). Artemisinin has been used in this way as an effective treatment for severe malaria in Vietnam (Arnold 1994).

In East Africa, quinine remains the standard treatment for severe malaria; a drug with high efficacy against the parasite at achievable in-vivo concentrations. Quinine does not prevent parasite sequestration or alter parasite clearance during the first 12 h of treatment. Against sensitive parasites, chloroquine was perhaps the ideal treatment for severe malaria when given by the parenteral route; inducing rapid clearance of parasites (White et al 1992). Unfortunately, this is no longer possible because of the high prevalence of chloroquine-resistant malaria in East Africa. Despite the use of effective treatment (quinine, together with appropriate supplementary clinical management—control of seizures, rehydration, control of metabolic acidosis), the mortality from severe disease remains high, at about 15%. Most of these deaths occur within 24 h of admission (Marsh et al 1995), which is a reflection of the rapid course of the disease in children, and also results from late presentation. On the Kenyan coast the pattern of "health seeking behaviour", which principally involves the mother, is becoming better understood. For fever, the initial recourse is to shop-bought medicine (usually chloroquine because it is cheap, and therefore stocked by village shops). Other definable symptoms may involve a visit to the local herbalist. If the child remains sick, or worsens, then hospital or health centre care is sought. Under the new arrangements for cost sharing in many African countries, this can be an expensive option for people who are essentially outside the cash economy. For these reasons, many children in Africa die at home, before reaching hospital (Greenwood et al 1987), or are admitted to hospital in a serious condition where the outcome may already be irreversible.

The treatment of non-severe falciparum malaria

As for severe malaria, the prime requirement for the successful treatment of non-severe, or outpatient malaria, is an effective, cheap drug, with a dosage regimen lasting no longer than three days. This last point is particularly important; if the drug works, the child will be getting better 24 to 48 h after the start of treatment. The mother will tend to reserve any remaining medication, which has been paid for, to treat the next similar episode (Foster 1991).

Chloroquine was, for about 40 years, the mainstay of outpatient malaria treatment. In East Africa, chloroquine-resistant falciparum malaria (CRFM) is now common in the high transmission areas, although still comparatively rare in some isolated regions, especially those such as Northern Turkana, characterized by less efficient mosquito vectors and a highly seasonal pattern of malaria (Clarke et al 1996). Unfortunately, these areas are few, accounting for a very small proportion of the malaria cases in the region. The antifolate antimalarial combinations, represented by pyrimethamine–sulphadoxine (PSD), remain generally effective treatments, although there are indications (both from theoretical considerations and from field studies) that this may be temporary. PSD is comparatively cheap, which is a very important consideration for almost all African countries. Although CRFM is widespread, most malaria infections still respond partially to chloroquine, with a rapid initial fall in peripheral parasitaemia, and clinical improvement which may be due in part to the potent antipyretic action of chloroquine. For these reasons, rather than a complete change from chloroquine to PSD, some centres find that a combination of the two drugs provides optimal treatment.

Drug Resistance and New Therapeutic Approaches

Several reports from South East Asia have described advantages of the artemisinin derivatives over quinine in the treatment of severe malaria. Quinine efficacy has been decreasing steadily in South East Asia for several years as a result of parasite resistance, and this may in part account for this observation, although the mechanisms of action of the two drugs are also dissimilar. In the treatment of patients with artemisinin compounds, two particular differences are apparent: the parasite clearance time is much shorter than with quinine and there is specific activity directed against the early ring stages.

Until very recently, it was thought that quinine exerted broad-spectrum activity against all the developmental blood stages of the parasite. This was shown not to be the case in a study at Kilifi which measured the viability of parasites ex-vivo from patients with non-severe malaria treated with different drugs. While the viability of parasites from quinine-treated, or PSD-treated patients remained > 90%, and no different to the pre-treatment samples for at least the first 24 h of therapy, in-vivo exposure to halofantrine for 6 h was sufficient to arrest parasite development. (Watkins et al 1993). We have recently shown that artemether (an oil-soluble artemisinin derivative formulated as an intramuscular injection) has a similar effect (Murphy et al 1995). Clearly, if artemether or a similar artemisinin derivative can arrest the development of young parasites to the stage at which they sequester, while at the same time rapidly reducing peripheral parasitaemia, these effects may translate into reduced mortality.

This was the rationale behind a multi-centre comparative trial of intramuscular artemether vs parenteral quinine, recently completed in Kenya, Malawi and Nigeria, in strictly defined cases of severe malaria, and with death as the endpoint. In all studies, parasite clearance was more rapid with artemether, but there was no difference in mortality between treatment groups (Murphy et al 1996). However, in the Kenyan study the concentrations of artemether and the major metabolite dihydroartemisinin which were achieved in-vivo varied widely between patients, and were significantly lower in patients with respiratory distress, a marker for metabolic acidosis. These are the sickest children and are often hypovolaemic with cool extremities, an indication of poor muscle perfusion (Murphy & Watkins, unpublished data). Although confirmation is needed, it is very likely that these patients did not absorb artemether, a poorly water-soluble drug, in sufficient amounts from the intramuscular site. More appropriate derivatives might be the water-soluble compounds sodium artesunate or artelinic acid, although these drugs are not yet available in Africa.

For the treatment of non-severe malaria, there is an urgent need to find alternatives to PSD. The long elimination half-life of this combination, which in the past was seen as a benefit because it protected the host from early re-infection, provides a potent mechanism for the selection of pyrimethamine-resistant parasites. In an area of continuous malaria transmission, the treated child is soon re-infected; residual physiological drug kills sensitive, but not resistant parasites. In a trial at Kilifi, 90% of new infections in the period 15 to 52 days following PSD treatment were pyrimethamine-resistant in-vitro, in contrast to a wild-type resistance prevalence of 15% (Watkins & Mosobo 1993). Further, the mutations in the parasite dihydrofolate reductase gene which govern resistance to individual antifolate drugs are known, and drug-specific. Work in Kilifi and Nairobi is addressing the efficacy and utility of chlorproguanil–dapsone (CPG–DDS) as an alternative to PSD. The new combination has the potential advantages of a short elimination half-life, and thus reduced selective pressure for resistance, and greater efficacy against pyrimethamine-resistant infections.

Another potentially useful antimalarial under investigation in Kenya is the benzonaphthyridine drug pyronaridine, a drug related structurally to both the acridine mepacrine, and to amodiaquine. Pyronaridine, synthesized in China in 1970 and used widely as an antimalarial drug in that country, is new to western medicine. Only one preliminary clinical trial has been conducted in Africa, but the results are encouraging. One hundred percent parasite clearance by day 7, with patients still parasite-free at 14 days, was achieved with pyronaridine, against infections which were mainly chloroquine-resistant (Ringwald et al1996). Work on pyronaridine is being actively pursued by WHO, since this drug may eventually present an effective and affordable replacement for chloroquine.

To ensure continued malaria control in East Africa there is an urgent need for new antimalarial drugs which will have a useful therapeutic life extending over at least 10 years, and which are affordable. If basic and operational research studies do not deliver effective new drugs in the near future, the outlook is bleak. Mefloquine, the drug which replaced PSD in South East Asia, is far too expensive to be purchased in adequate amounts in Africa, and the same consideration applies to all the current alternative treatments, even if demand forces price reductions. It is unlikely that the available alternative drugs will ever become cheap enough to ensure that all cases of malaria are treated. In this scenario, an alarming rise in malaria-related morbidity and mortality is likely to occur in the future. Ways must be found to address and solve this problem.

References

Arnold, K. (1994) Early treatment of malaria in the community using artemisinin – hope or hazard? Trans. R. Soc. Trop. Med. Hyg. 88 (Suppl. 1): 47–49

Clarke, D., Odialla, H., Ouma, J., Kenny, V., MacCabe, R., Rapuoda, B., Watkins, W. M. (1996) A malariometric survey in Turkana District, Kenya: chemosensitivity of in-vivo Plasmodium falciparum infections and identity of the vector. Trans. R. Soc. Trop. Med. Hyg. 90: 302–304

English, M., Crawley, J., Waruiru, C., Mwangi, I., Amukoiye, E., Marsh, K. (1996) Cerebral malaria is not an homogenous clinical syndrome. 17th African Health Sciences Congress, Kenya Medical Research Institute, Nairobi, Kenya, 5–9th Feb. (abstract)

Foster, S. D. (1991) Pricing, distribution and use of antimalarial drugs. Bull. World Health Organisation 69: 349–363

Greenwood, B. M., Bradley, A. K., Greenwood, A. M., Byass, P., Jammeh, K., Marsh, K., Tulloch, S., Oldfield, F. J. S., Hayes, R. (1987) Mortality and morbidity from malaria among children in a rural area of the Gambia. Trans. R. Soc. Trop. Med. Hyg. 81: 478–486

Marsh, K., Forster, D., Waruiru, C., Mwangi, I., Winstanley, M., Marsh, V., Newton, C., Winstanley, P. A., Warn, P., Peshu, N., Pasvol, G., Snow, R. W. (1995) Indicators of life-threatening malaria in African children. N. Engl. J. Med. 332: 1399–1404

Murphy, S. A., Watkins, W. M., Bray, P., Lowe, B., Winstanley, P. A., Marsh, K. (1995) Parasite viability during treatment of severe falciparum malaria: differential effects of artemether and quinine. Am. J. Trop. Med. Hyg. 53: 303–305

Murphy, S., English, M., Waruiru, C., Mwangi, I., Amukoye, E., Crawley, J., Newton, C., Winstanley, P. A., Peshu, N., Marsh, K. (1996) An open randomised trial of artemether versus quinine in the treatment of cerebral malaria in African children. Trans. R. Soc. Trop. Med. Hyg. 90: 298–302

Pavitt, N. (1989) Kenya: the first explorers. Aurum Press Ltd, London

Ringwald, P., Bickii, J., Basco, L. (1996) Randomised trial of pyronaridine versus chloroquine for acute uncomplicated falciparum malaria in Africa. Lancet 347: 24–28

Waller, D., Krishna, S., Crawley, J., Miller, K., Nosten, F., Chapman, D., ter Kuile, F. O., Craddock, C., Berry, C., Holloway, P. A. H., Brewster, D., Greenwood, B. M., White, N. J. (1995). Clinical features and outcome of severe malaria in Gambian children. Clin. Infect. Dis. 21: 577–587

Warrell, D. A. (1993) Treatment and prevention of malaria. In: Gilles, H. M., Warrell, D. A. (eds) Essential Malariology. 3rd edn, Edward Arnold, London, p. 183

Watkins, W. M., Mosobo, M. (1993) Treatment of Plasmodium falciparum malaria with pyrimethamine-sulfadoxine: selective pressure for resistance is a function of long elimination half life. Trans. R. Soc. Trop. Med. Hyg. 87: 75–78

Watkins, W. M., Woodrow, C., Marsh, K. (1993) Falciparum malaria: differential effects of antimalarial drugs on ex vivo parasite viability during the critical early phase of therapy. Am. J. Trop. Med. Hyg. 49: 106–112

White, N. J., Ho, M. (1992) The pathophysiology of malaria. Adv. Parasitol 31: 84–173

White, N. J., Krishna, S. (1989) Treatment of malaria: some considerations and limitations of the current methods of assessment. Trans. R. Soc. Trop. Med. Hyg. 83: 767–777

White, N. J., Chapman, D., Watt, G. (1992) The effect of multiplication and synchronicity on the vascular distribution of parasites in falciparum malaria. Trans. R. Soc. Trop. Med. Hyg. 86: 590–597

Winstanley, P. A., Watkins, W. M., Newton, C. R. J. C., Nevill, C., Mberu, E., Warn, P. A., Waruira, C. M., Mwangi, I. N., Warrell, D. A., Maesh, K. (1992) The disposition of oral and intramuscular pyrimethamine/sulfadoxine in Kenyan children with high parasitaemia but clinically non-severe falciparum malaria. Br. J. Clin. Pharmacol. 33: 143–148

World Health Organization, Division of Control of Tropical Diseases. (1990) Severe and complicated malaria. Second Edition. Trans. R. Soc. Trop. Med. Hyg. 84 (Suppl. 2): 1–65

J. Pharm. Pharmacol. 1997, 49 (Suppl. 2): 13–16

Malaria in Southern Africa

P. V. ROLLASON

Hillside Pharmacy, Hillside Shopping Centre, Box 9002, Hillside, Bulawayo, Zimbabwe

I would wish you to see malaria through the eyes of one who deals with the disease every day of the week. The situation of a community pharmacist in a malarious area is very different from that of a researcher, or even a medical practitioner/prescriber. The disease presents itself to a community pharmacist as patients in a scare situation, bedevilled by confused utterances; scared because 600 people died of it in Zimbabwe in 1995; confused by so much differing advice on offer by everyone from the Professor to the next door neighbour. I will try to clarify the existing situation of the disease as seen in Southern Africa.

Vector Control

Urban areas, in some cases cities of a million or more people, are generally controlled at the start of the season by residual insecticide spraying undertaken by the local authority and concentrated on standing waters. Most of these major urban areas are situated on the highveld above 1000 metres altitude, which means in this part of Africa there is a very low risk of malaria. It is acknowledged that the altitude parameter of anophelene breeding varies as one moves nearer to the equator. In rural areas and especially those below 1000 metres, residual insecticide spraying is normally undertaken by central governments. Even when DDT was used, this presented no environmental hazard as the spraying was confined to dwellings both inside and outside. As a measure of its success, when the government runs out of money (far too frequently) and spraying at the beginning of the rainy season is reduced, morbidity and, distressingly mortality more than doubles. There has been encouragement for the greater use of bed nets, pre-soaked with pyrethrins where possible but this has not been very successful. It is general policy in Zimbabwe and its surrounding countries not to supply any form of chemoprophylaxis to constant dwellers in rural malarious areas. These people who are challenged daily with infected vectors, are regarded as being partial immunes, probably with a similar degree of success as would be achieved by most preventive drug regimes. But of course, urban high-veld dwellers visiting low-veld malarious areas need a preventive drug, and this is where a problem immediately arises. For example, a peasant family lives in a low-veld malarious area, Tjolotjo, but the father works at a factory on the high-veld in Bulawayo 100 km away. The family are partial immunes, but he is not. When he goes to visit them once in three or four months, he is advised to take his malaria tablets. But he says: "I do not need medicine; I am not sick. My wife and children do not take anything so why must I" He takes nothing and he gets malaria. Added to that, the confused story of prophylaxis and the various regimes on offer makes for a very difficult situation. There is also another point that should be mentioned: that of communication and knowledge of language and local customs.

We are experiencing more and more "Commuter malaria".

Where I live on the high-veld in what is regarded as a non-malarious area, no prophylaxis is advocated and generally not used. However there are more and more cases of malaria being contracted in these areas, contrary to expectations. These are mosquitoes that go "walk-about". They travel in from malarious to non-malarious areas on buses, trains and bicycles, and do their damage on arrival. We had a fatal case of cerebral falciparum about three years ago in Bulawayo. The mosquito had hitched a ride in a boat trailer of some people who had been having a holiday on Lake Kariba, in the Zambezi valley. The trailer was parked on arrival home; the mosquito escaped and bit the lady who lived next door. She had not been out of the town for over two years, and yet she died from malaria because it had neither been suspected nor had it been thought of geographically for diagnosis. Another lady who collapsed seemingly from general malaise and possible malnutrition was given a routine blood test and surprisingly malaria was found. She was treated with chloroquine and fully recovered. The offending mosquito apparently came into town wrapped in the blankets of one of her employees returning to work after spending the Christmas holidays in a malarious area.

Treatment and Diagnosis

Probably of prime importance, however, is malaria treatment per se. I, of course, can only relate my own region's circumstances. Up as far as the Zambezi River, resistance to chloroquine, although known and documented, is generally isolated and not too significant. In fact chloroquine resistance is greatly over-estimated. Why should this be so? The answer to this vexed question (and I am sure this applies to many other parts of the world) is inaccurate diagnosis. Chloroquine is, as we know the drug of choice and is still remarkably effective. It is widely used, easily available and cheap. Some years ago it was decided to make chloroquine freely available to people especially in rural areas through local general stores so that when they felt that they were succumbing to malaria, they could easily buy treatment close to home. The normally recommended dose was well publicized and encouraged. It all went wrong. The people bought the chloroquine, but usually only two tablets to cure a headache or a hangover or conversely, a massive quantity to provoke an abortion. The amount used for the legitimate treatment of malaria was negligible. This has been partly overcome by confining the product to sale only in original packs of ten tablets, but obviously this is not the answer.

The only place where accurate diagnosis of malaria can occur is in towns where there is a laboratory with a good microscope and above all a well trained technologist to read and interpret the blood slides. In most parts of the area this just doesn't happen. There was a World Health Organization (WHO) plan a couple of years ago to obtain some 2000 microscopes, to send them out to the rural areas to increase diagnostic efficiency. There was no one to read the slides, even if they could have been prepared, there was no electricity for illumination and no microscopes working—they were either broken, stolen or sold. All this serves therefore to highlight a system that is prevalent throughout—presumptive diagnosis. This means in essence, that when a person feels unwell even with minor symptoms and has been in a malarious area, chloroquine is given in a full dose regime. If that person recovers, fine; it was malaria and has been dealt with. But so often he does not respond. Is the inference to be that chloroquine failed? Not at all—he has not had malaria but more than likely influenza, diarrhoea, dysentery or, particularly, tick fever. Fortunately chloroquine seems to have few side effects in an otherwise uncompromized person, and even skin itching although known, is nothing like as severe in my part of Africa as has been encountered in parts of West Africa. So, we have a system of basic misdiagnosis and this is very often classified as an example of chloroquine-resistant malaria. In fact the figures given for such resistance are so false that they are, in my estimation, about 50%. I have heard of quotes from other sources that the figures may be as high as 60% wrong. There is also another reason for confusion. Hardly any local medical practitioners and even some epidemiologists know what chloroquine resistance means. They are not aware of R1, R2 and R3 resistance, let alone the more recent WHO parameters of resistance estimation.

Diagnosis therefore is the kingpin of malaria containment. And there is much hope in this direction. The incidence of different malarial strains in Zimbabwe and Southern Africa generally is estimated roughly as *P. falciparum* 98%, *P. malariae* 1·5%, *P. ovale* 0·5% and *P. vivax* nil. The diagnostic system that measures the histidine rich protein of falciparum invasion by means of a dipstick procedure is therefore most valuable. I introduced this into Zimbabwe last year, and the manufacturers donated a set of 100 tests for trial. In the city of Bulawayo I worked with general practitioners, and when they had a case of suspected malaria, they telephoned me, and I went immediately to their surgery and did the test with them on the spot (an unusual role for a city pharmacist, but one that paid dividends!). Every diagnosis was deliberately confirmed by blood slides which could require a day or more to produce a result, but every single one was confirmed. The point here is that every positive case was commenced on treatment at once and results were 100% successful. Negative diagnosis required the doctor to think again and in every case another disease was found and then adequately treated. After a number of tests done this way, I gave the remainder to the local laboratory who conducted them for the general practitioners at no cost. They then purchased more, and the service was installed until (luckily at the end of the season) supplies from the manufacturer ran out. The USA could not cope with demand! There is now also an even cheaper ICT Rapid Malaria Test and, like the Parasight F test mentioned above, is specific for *P. falciparum* and these are just what we need. There should be just such a simple diagnostic system installed at every health clinic, every mobile health centre, and even with village health workers. Malaria would thus be much more accurately and efficiently dealt with, and a lot of unnecessary treatment and drug use avoided. Incidentally, the Parasight F test can even be done by someone who is illiterate, and takes less then ten minutes.

Coming now to the classic situation of *P. falciparum* malaria, what treatment policy is followed in Southern Africa? Chloroquine is still our number one drug. The drug of second choice and beloved by travellers from overseas to carry as a "stand-by" is pyrimethamine and sulphadoxine combination. The third line of treatment is mefloquine or halofantrine—the former not much used, the latter used generally successfully but now less popular because of its erratic absorption and its known cardiac side-effects. Quinine is still high on the list and used quite extensively. Most recently, artemisinin and derivatives, usually in the form of artemether injection, is being used by some doctors, generally with excellent results. So what problems do we have? With chloroquine, very few. We do know of resistance, we know where it occurs in isolated pockets but as yet these do not appear significant. We have found nausea and vomiting a problem especially when the initial dose of 600 mg base is taken but this is almost always overcome if administered with a glucose drink. Pyrimethamine–sulphadoxine is unquestionably an effective treatment, but has a complicating factor: after administration of the usual three tablet dose the patients symptoms usually improve quite soon—in 36 h or less—but when blood slides are taken parasitaemia remains higher than expected. Many practitioners are not aware that in the case of this drug the parasite load is reduced rather slowly, so they panic and rush to give quinine with all its nasty side effects, basically unnecessarily. Mefloquine is not much used for treatment, for no valid reason except perhaps expense. And as I mentioned, artemisinin is very successful in recalcitrant cases, a heavy parasite load and in the distressing escalation of cerebral malaria. Resistances to quinine and others, including mefloquine and halofantrine have not been recorded. Incidentally, very few doctors and even fewer patients are aware that cerebral malaria is as a result of either undiagnosed or inadequately treated *P. falciparum* malaria, and regard it as a special, different, fatal disease.

Prophylaxis

Malaria is not a notifiable disease in terms of law and therefore incidences and geographical disposition can only be assessed by positive visits and voluntary reports. The Zimbabwe government has a research laboratory in Harare that concerns itself among other things with malaria, and there is a malaria unit within the Ministry of Health and Child Welfare. They both work in conjunction with the WHO sub-regional office in the same city.

In 1994 I was awarded an F.I.P., scholarship to research malaria incidence, treatment and prevention in Southern Africa, I concentrated on four countries—South Africa, Namibia, Botswana and Zimbabwe. South Africa is well involved in malaria work, and a special unit under the Medical Research Council employs more than twenty people concerned mainly in researching chloroquine resistance. Under the direction of Dr Brian Sharpe, they are also constructing malaria maps for the regions and I have been able to supply him with the Zimbabwe component. Namibia and Botswana have no research but generally follow WHO guidelines. Zimbabwe does more, although it does not have a specific biological research laboratory. Where treatment is concerned there is little difference within the four countries, drug availability being the main limiting factor. However, where prophylaxis and particularly advice on prophylaxis is concerned there is utmost confusion. I must mention here South Africa's policy of recommending mefloquine as the main preventive drug to be used and registering it only for that purpose. It may not be used for treatment. A doctors prescription is required, costs are phenomenally high, and in spite of what the texts and promotion says, the incidence of unacceptable side-effects, especially in the first few weeks, is very high. This has, furthermore, led to a bad reputation for the drug among the lay public, and more importantly to poor compliance and thus increased risk. Contrary to this, we in Zimbabwe have used pyrimethamine-dapsone for over twenty years as our main preventative with excellent results and no known single case of agranulocytosis or resistance has been recorded. I was delighted to see acknowledgement of our use of this combination in the March 1995 edition of the British National Formulary. Proguanil and chloroquine is still used occasionally as prophylactic treatment but only where a patient shows a sulphonamide allergy to dapsone. Side-effects from this universally recommended regime of proguanil and chloroquine

are much higher than generally acknowledged. This leads to poor compliance. Any patient who has to take sixteen tablets a week when he is not ill and then feels terrible, is not very likely to continue. Incidentally, whatever regime of prophylaxis is used, we advocate continuance for four weeks after leaving a malarious area, as generally we have no *P. vivax.* I found that Botswana was only recommending two weeks—I think they have now changed.

Titrating the dose of any drug for children is always somewhat hazardous. Age is the usual measurement but children vary tremendously in size and weight for age. Thus there is a tendency to marginally overdose. In one part of my country where the population is concentrated under one employer, pyrimethamine-dapsone is administered every Monday. On that day quite a number of children go blue from slight dapsone overdosage but it doesn't matter and simply acts as a proof that the dose has been taken. The origin of "Blue Monday" perhaps? I have records from the hospital that administers this whole area and even during this last bad season not one employee had malaria.

There is little doubt that in practice, the success of malaria

Table 1. Typical problems in malaria prophylaxis arising from case studies.

Problem	Answer
During a bad season should one increase the preventive dose of pyrimethamine-dapsone to one tablet every five days rather than the usual seven days?	No. The difference in serum levels between five and seven days is only about 2% and compliance on a five day dosage is likely to be nil.
Should one add chloroquine to pyrimethamine-dapsone during the bad season to get better protection?	Not a bad idea, but the dose of chloroquine should be taken when the effectiveness of pyrinethamine dapsone is running out, that is five days later, and compliance is likely to be very poor.
A patient has an allergy to sulphonamides and seemingly to chloroquine, reacts badly to proguanil, and has minor psychiatric problems treated with tri-cyclic anti-depressants. What preventative would he take?	Possibly tetracycline i.e. doxycycline 100 mg day^{-1}.
A woman is three months pregnant and has to visit a malarious area. What must she take?	Pyrimethamine-dapsone all through pregnancy. She should also have a folic acid supplement, 5 mg daily, and we suggest also 250 mg vitamin C.
An epileptic lady is treated regularly with phenobarbitone and clonazepam. What preventative should she take?	We suggest pyrimethamine-dapsone, but starting four weeks before entering a malarious area to allow time for dose adjustment of her epileptic drugs, (it was found necessary to slightly increase her dose of clonazepam).
A child aged about eleven presented every few weeks with recurrent falciparum malaria was treated in turn with chloroquine, quinine, and halofantrine; but why the recurrence?	The most likely explanation was a constant re-challenge as he lived on the borders of a malarious area, but there is also the possibility of inadequate dosage through considerable vomiting that was not compensated for.
An elderly Zimbabwean lived back in the UK for ten years then returned to Africa. She brought proguanil and chloroquine which she took although she was in a non-malarious area and did not need to. She developed very bad mouth sores and aphthous ulcers.	We took her off all medication and she was fine. Although she had lived here previously she was scared because of all the stories she had heard in the UK about Southern Africa.

(In passing, no inoculations whatever are needed for travellers to Zimbabwe and nearby countries unless coming through Zaire when yellow fever is good. We had one poor man who had been bludgeoned by his doctor into having eight different inoculations—including rabies—all unnecessary!).

chemoprophylaxis depends on compliance with the medication dosage provided. Many people, especially travellers, carry stand-by medication when visiting malarious areas. Upon feeling unwell the medication is taken and all too frequently incorrectly. For example, a course of three tablets of pyrmethmine-sulphadoxine will be carried for just such an eventuality, but the person feels only a little ill, but suspects malaria—is not sure—so takes one tablet just in case. Similar scenarios occur with chloroquine. Money also plays an important part: in Zimbabwe, pyrimethamine-dapsone costs the patient about ZIM$16·00 for 20 tablets—enough for five weeks prevention for four people. Proguanil–chloroquine, to cover the same number of people for the same period, would cost about ZIM$650·00; mefloquine would be ZIM$945·00—40 and 60 times the cost of pyrimethamine-dapsone, respectively! Which would you choose, given that the results are reasonably equivalent? Especially if you live there and have a monthly income of abound ZIM$1000·00 per month. Perhaps now you can see the popularity of pyrimethamine–dapsone as our malaria preventative.

Following along this line, I wonder what your opinion would be of a general practice doctor who himself lives in a seasonal malarious area and recommends to his patient no chemoprophylaxis at all. He maintains it suppresses the disease and masks its diagnosis. He has limited diagnostic facilities and certainly no dipstick test. Table 1 poses a number of problems encountered in malaria prophylaxis and are all case studies—actual occurrences that we have had to deal with.

I have not mentioned the possibility of a vaccine which so many of you are deeply concerned with. There is good reason. It will, with all respect, have very little impact on us at all. With a population of about 11 million variously exposed to malaria, no one or no country will be able to periodically vaccinate everyone against malaria by virtue of practicality and finance. As far as we can assess the situation the vaccine will be of value to the fairly well-off traveller as cover for a short period.

Conclusions

In summary, Southern Africa has a bad enough malaria situation, but chloroquine still works and other drugs are available and effective. There is much more interaction between neighbouring countries now than ever before and are working now on a malaria 6-year plan, possibly financed by Australia, to co-ordinate work on this disease and its containment. This scheme will be centred on Harare, Zimbabwe.

I was, however, interested in news recently of an idea to genetically engineer anophelene mosquitos so that they give a bite which introduces a protective protein, and hence limits the disease. The idea of millions of flying vaccinations is mind boggling. The Swiss have recently come out with a little electric device which sends out a supersonic noise that repels mosquitos. But when questioned as to what happened with anopheles which do not buzz, and therefore may not react accordingly, they were not quite sure. We always tell our visitors that the malarial mosquito does not buzz, has stripes or spots, sticks her backside in the air to bite and only does so at sunset or later. So if they are having a sundowner drink and come across such an animal which they cannot see or hear, they should certainly kill it! And the best malaria preventive of all is gin and tonic. The tonic water provides quinine and if you have enough, the gin results in alcoholic mosquitos who get so drunk they don't know what they are doing!

J. Pharm. Pharmacol. 1997, 49 (Suppl. 2): 17–19

Coping With Malaria While We Wait for a Vaccine

PETER WINSTANLEY

w>Department of Pharmacology and Therapeutics, New Medical Building, University of Liverpool, Liverpool L69 3BX, UK.

Malaria remains as much a scourge as ever. Of the four species of plasmodia capable of infecting man it is *Plasmodium falciparum* with which we have most problems because this species not only causes life-threatening illness but has also developed resistance to most classes of antimalarial drugs. Therefore, it is falciparum malaria that will be discussed here. Furthermore, although *P. falciparum* is a problem in much of the tropics, most cases and associated deaths are seen in sub-Saharan Africa: about 12 million cases and 1·2 million deaths annually (Anon. 1995). Most African nations are not only faced with many pressing healthcare problems (tuberculosis, diarrhoeal diseases and HIV to name but three) but also have extremely hard-pressed healthcare resources. Consequently, falciparum malaria in Africa will be the main focus of the present summary.

Although eradication of malaria was once a goal, the main target of control programmes over the last two decades has been reduction of the appalling mortality and morbidity figures cited above. Unfortunately it seems very likely that, over the next two decades, the trend is likely to worsen under the influence of global warming (and hence the possibility that malaria prevalence rates may rise) and the inexorable spread of multi-drug-resistant *P. falciparum*: it may be that we shall count ourselves lucky if we can hold mortality figures as they are, let alone reduce them.

Some of the Available Strategies

Plasmodium parasitaemia, particularly with *P. falciparum* is extremely (although variably) prevalent throughout tropical Africa: in parts of east Africa, for example, the prevalence rate can be as high as 80% in children at certain times of the year. Typically, only a proportion of children with parasitaemia develop symptoms and only a small proportion of these become severely ill or die (Marsh et al 1995). Africa is vast, and the epidemiology of clinical malaria is extremely complex; it is influenced to a large degree by factors like: variation in climate (mainly rainfall patterns); the biting habits of the predominant vector (usually the *Anopheles gambiae* complex); the culture and beliefs of the population, and their healthcare-seeking behaviour; availability and funding of healthcare; and access to means of travel. This, of course, is not an exhaustive list. Clearly, the relative importance of each factor in each geographical location would need to be addressed in a systematic manner for interventions to be chosen logically, but such data are lamentably incomplete and our attempts at control remain sub-optimal.

Certainly the "best" way to reduce malaria mortality figures for an average population in sub-Saharan Africa would be to tackle poverty, but more immediately-available targets include: reduction in transmission; mass chemoprophylaxis; effective treatment of non-severe disease (mainly based in out-patient departments); and improved treatment of severe disease (based in in-patient facilities).

Reduced transmission

Female *Anopheles* mosquitoes bite at night, and sleeping under nets reduces transmission. Herodotus, describing his travels around the Ancient World (The Histories), is the earliest author that I have been able to find who mentions the use of bednets (in the Egyptian delta) to prevent the nuisance of nocturnal insect bites. Bednets have had an established rational role in malaria prevention for about a century. More recently, dipping the nets in permethrin insecticide has been shown to be an effective means of reducing mortality in malaria-exposed African populations (Nevill et al 1996). The results of such work have been impressive. However, for such an intervention to be successful on a national scale, a number of factors would need to be addressed including adequate organization (including distribution, regular dipping and maintenance), adequate infrastructure (e.g. roads, networks of verbal/written communication) and adequate funding. Furthermore, several possible disadvantages will need to be considered before the intervention becomes generally adopted, such as diversion of funds from other national healthcare budgets (will supra-national funds be made available?) and the effects of interruption of the program on malaria mortality (will prevention of parasite transmission eradicate the development of immunity?)

Mass chemoprophylaxis

Chemoprophylaxis for foreign visitors to high transmission areas is standard practice, but such subjects are exposed for a finite period (commonly less than 4 weeks) and are able to bear the cost themselves. In contrast, African populations can expect to remain exposed to transmission throughout their lives and usually are unable to afford long-term antimalarial drugs. Certainly, the population acquires partial immunity to local strains of the parasite, so that continual exposure makes severe illness unlikely, but high-risk sub-groups remain. Furthermore, this partial immunity is bought at a terrible cost in childhood deaths. The high-risk sub-groups, particularly pregnant women, can usually be offered chemoprophylaxis because they self-present, making logistics manageable, they are at risk for a finite period and the programme can be kept cost-effective if the drugs are inexpensive (and costs are generally met by the State). However the scale of offering chemoprophylaxis to the whole under-5 age group is much larger: the pros and cons have been reviewed by Greenwood (1984).

Treatment of severe disease

Only a proportion of children with symptomatic falciparum

malaria go on to develop a severe or fatal illness (most commonly cerebral malaria, severe anaemia and metabolic acidosis—the three groups are not mutually exclusive), and so it may seem logical to concentrate resources trying to save these few. A moment's reflection reveals the difficulties of this approach, in that only a proportion of severe disease reaches hospital or health-care outposts (the proportion is, obviously, very variable depending on the proximity and standard of care offered; we usually have few data on proportions of malaria deaths occurring at home). Also, high-dependency care is, relatively, very expensive. Nevertheless, this is not to say that no attempt should be made to target this group: Marsh et al (1991) have calculated that a large proportion of severely ill children in their area are treated in hospital. Certainly the provision of simple measures, including administration of an effective parenteral antimalarial drug, dipstick measurement of blood sugar and 50% glucose, and safe blood transfusion, would save many lives and would probably be cost-effective in comparison with other interventions. Surprising though it may seem these, apparently basic, requirements are not universally available.

Further lives would probably be saved by provision of the following: increased nursing and medical staffing; diagnostic bacteriology (serious bacterial infections including bacteraemia and meningitis may co-exist with malaria); and a greater range of relatively sophisticated drugs (including parenteral anti-epileptics and newer antibiotics). However, these provisions are relatively expensive. Furthermore, it should be borne in mind that even when treatment budgets and staffing levels are high the mortality rate for cerebral malaria falls no lower than around 10% (Marsh et al 1995). Thus, ever increasing expenditure in this area could be expected to make only a limited improvement in mortality figures. Anathema though it might be to the practising physician (and I am one), when faced with difficult choices, planners may conclude that more lives could be saved by spending money in other areas of malaria control.

On the other hand, which parenteral antimalarial drug to choose for severe falciparum malaria (and how to give it) has received much attention in the last few years. If the simple process of changing drug could be shown to save lives, then this would probably be an affordable intervention. Quinine is currently the drug of first-choice in Africa, not because of its great potency, but because it is reliable (resistance has not been encountered). Unfortunately, quinine does not kill circulating parasites (Watkins et al 1991) which remain available to sequester in deep structures, possibly worsening outcome. The artemisinin-derivatives, on the other hand, have early effects on circulating ring-forms (Murphy et al 1995) and might be expected to reduce mortality. Unfortunately, randomized trials in Kenya (Murphy et al 1996) and elsewhere have failed to show such an effect on mortality, although artemether was at least as effective as quinine. A number of unanswered questions remain, including: what effect would artemisinin-deriv-atives have on mortality if given intravenously (artemether is given intramuscularly, and there are some concerns over its absorption) and does the use of artemisinins lower mortality in those children with uncomplicated disease, who may be at high risk of developing severe malaria (e.g. the very young, the anaemic and those with high circulating parasite loads)?

It is, of course, essential that fundamental research continues into the mechanisms (both molecular and pathophysiological) which underlie the development of severe disease. Improvement in understanding the problem will surely help us to tackle it more effectively.

Treatment of uncomplicated malaria

Throughout much of sub-Saharan Africa uncomplicated falciparum malaria is among the commonest causes of hospital attendance. Another way of looking at the same statement is that most cases of symptomatic falciparum malaria seek treatment: they may not necessarily attend hospital (distances may be too great and the waiting times too long) but may obtain their drugs from local shops (Mwenesi et al 1995). This group represents a self-selected opportunity for intervention. In practice, of course, treatment of symptomatic disease has long been the main malaria control measure employed in Africa. In my opinion this intervention is set to retain its pre-eminent place—so long as effective, practicable and affordable drugs are available. The importance of drug cost cannot be over-emphasized.

What follows is not meant to be a review of the Clinical Pharmacology of antimalarial drugs, but rather an attempt to put their usefulness into context in an African setting.

Chloroquine. In view of almost ubiquitous resistance throughout Africa, chloroquine cannot be recommended for non-immune patients with uncomplicated falciparum malaria. However, in many malaria-endemic countries, chloroquine remains the drug of first-choice. This is the product of extremely difficult health-care decisions on deployment of scarce resources—malaria is only one of many health-care problems, and even pyrimethamine–sulphadoxine (PM–SD) costs more than chloroquine.

Quinine. One might imagine that, faced with chloroquine-resistance, reversion to oral quinine therapy would be an obvious solution. Unfortunately quinine has the following major disadvantages: it is considerably more expensive than chloroquine; it must be given several times daily for at least 5 days; and it tastes appalling in the liquid suspensions needed for paediatric use. In consequence, although quinine is used for uncomplicated disease, availability is limited and compliance is poor.

Mefloquine. This synthetic drug has structural similarities to quinine. It is effective against *P falciparum* strains resistant to chloroquine and PM–SD, and is therefore extensively used in Indochina. Although mefloquine is marketed in some African countries, and is very potent against local *P. falciparum* strains, it is little used because it is unaffordable by the vast bulk of the population.

Halofantrine. Halofantrine is effective against many strains of *P falciparum* resistant to chloroquine, PM–SD and mefloquine, and is used extensively in parts of Indochina. Like mefloquine, halofantrine is rarely used in Africa because of its high cost.

Artemisinin and derivatives. Semi-synthetic artemisinin-derivatives are available in oral (and rectal) formulation, and can be expected to be effective in an African setting. Their cost, which will be the critical determinant of their utility, is unclear at present but is likely to be relatively high. In contrast, artemisinin itself is cheaper to produce (it has merely to be isolated from plant material and formulated; no derivatization is required) and is extensively used for this reason in Vietnam. It is possible that oral/rectal artemisinin preparations may prove practicable for uncomplicated malaria in some parts of Africa, although the long treatment course needed to prevent recrudescence (5 days) is potentially a major disadvantage.

Pyrimethamine–sulphadoxine and other antifolate combinations. PM–SD is cheap, practicable (only one dose is needed) and highly effective in much of Africa. Not surprisingly this combination is fast becoming the drug of first-choice for uncomplicated disease. In much of Indochina, where parasites are often resistant to both PM and SD, PM–SD is clinically useless. Such resistance is unusual in Africa at the moment, but is confidently awaited and, unless an affordable replacement is available, the impact on mortality figures may well be major.

PM–SD is eliminated slowly (half-lives of 81 and 116 h respectively), which provides welcome chemoprophylaxis after treatment, but also favours the selection of parasites resistant to PM (Watkins & Mosobo 1993) and possibly also to SD. Rapidly-eliminated antifolate drugs are likely to exert less resistance selection pressure than PM–SD. Furthermore, *P. falciparum* resistant to PM retains sensitivity to other dihydrofolate reductase inhibitors. Chlorcycloguanil (the active metabolite of chlorproguanil) combined with dapsone is more potent in-vitro than PM–SD (Winstanley et al 1995) and is eliminated rapidly (half-lives lives of 12·6 and 24·5 h respectively). Consequently, our teams in Kenya and Malawi hypothesize that chlorproguanil–dapsone is at least as effective as PM–SD, that it exerts less selective pressure for resistance and that it will retain efficacy as PM–SD failure emerges. We are currently in the process of testing these hypotheses.

Conclusions

Ninety percent of global malaria mortality occurs in Africa. The absolute numbers of malaria deaths is likely to rise in the next decade. Insecticide-dipped bednets reduce malaria mortality, but the long-term sustainability of this intervention on a national scale has not been proved. Provision of antimalarial drugs for uncomplicated malaria is likely to remain among the more effective forms of malaria control.

Chloroquine is no longer reliable and pyrimethamine–sulphadoxine is the only affordable alternative presently available. However, resistance to pyrimethamine–sulphadoxine is likely to emerge within the next 10 years.

Effective, safe and affordable drugs for falciparum malaria are needed urgently.

References

Anon. (1995) Twelfth programme report of the UNDP-World Bank-WHO Special Programme for Research and Training in Tropical Diseases (TDR). World Health Organization, Geneva

Greenwood, B. M. (1984) The impact of malaria chemoprophylaxis on the immune status of Africans. Bull. WHO 62: 69–75

Marsh, K., Newton, C. J. R. C., Winstanley, P. A., Kirkham, F. J. (1991) Clinical malaria: new problems in patient management. In: Targett, G. A. T. (ed.) Malaria, Waiting for the Vaccine. Wiley, UK

Marsh, K., Forster, D., Waruiru, C., Mwangi, I., Winstanley, M., Marsh, V., Newton, C., Winstanley, P., Warn, P., Peshu, N. (1995) Indicators of life-threatening malaria in African children. N. Engl. J. Med. 332: 1399–404

Murphy, S., Watkins, W. M., Bray, P., Lowe, B., Winstanley, P. A., Marsh, K. (1995) Parasite viability during the treatment of severe falciparum malaria: differential effects of artemether and quinine. Am. J. Trop. Med. Hyg. 53: 303–305

Murphy, S., English, M., Waruiru, C., Mwangi, I., Amukoye, E., Crawley, J., Newton, C., Winstanley, P. A., Peshu, N., Marsh, K. (1996) An open randomised trial of artemether versus quinine in the treatment of cerebral malaria in African children. Trans. R. Soc. Trop. Med. Hyg. 90: 298–301

Mwenesi, H., Harpham, T., Snow, R. W. (1995) Child malaria treatment among mothers in Kenya. Social Science Med. 49: 1271–1277

Nevill, C. G., Some, E. S., Mungala, V. O., Mutemi, W., New, L., Marsh, K., Lengeler, C., Snow, R. W. (1996) Insecticide-treated bednets reduce mortality and severe morbidity from malaria among children on the Kenyan coast. Trop. Med. Int. Health 1: 139–146

Watkins, W. M., Mosobo, M. (1993) Treatment of *Plasmodium falciparum* malaria with pyrimethamine and sulphadoxine: a selective pressure for resistance in a function of long elimination half-life. Trans. R. Soc. Trop. Med. Hyg. 87: 75–79

Watkins, W. M., Woodrow, C., Marsh, K. (1991) Falciparum malaria: differential effects of antimalarial drugs on ex vivo parasite viability during the critical early phase of therapy. Am. J. Trop. Med. Hyg. 49: 106–112

Winstanley, P. A., Mberu, E. K., Szwandt, I. S. F., Breckenridge, A. M., Watkins, W. M. (1995) The *in-vitro* activity of novel antifolate drug combinations against *Plasmodium falciparum* and human granulocyte colony-forming-units. Antimicrob. Agents Chemother. 39: 948–952

J. Pharm. Pharmacol. 1997, 49 (Suppl. 2): 21–27

Malaria Vaccines: Current Status and Future Prospects

ELEANOR RILEY

Institute of Cell, Animal and Population Biology, Ashworth Laboratories, University of Edinburgh, Edinburgh, EH9 3JT, UK

Malaria is a mosquito-borne protozoal disease which is endemic in many tropical and subtropical regions of the world. *Plasmodium falciparum* and *Plasmodium vivax* are the most common species of human malaria and the most pathogenic. *P. vivax* causes the classical recurrent/relapsing febrile illness which is widely recognized as typical of malaria; although it causes severe morbidity, it is rarely fatal. *P. falciparum*, on the other hand, presents a much more variable picture. Symptoms may be severe or deceptively mild but the disease is fatal in approximately 1% of cases. Death may follow an acute infection (endotoxic shock or cerebral malaria) or may be the result of severe anaemia following chronic infection. The World Health Organization (WHO) estimates that up to 300 million cases and 3 million deaths occur worldwide each year. Malaria has traditionally been controlled either by preventing contact between the mosquito vector and human host or by chemotherapy (as discussed elsewhere in this volume). The only significant breakthrough in malaria control in the last decade has been the introduction of pyrethroid-impregnated bed nets: in controlled trials, treated bed nets have been shown to reduce *P. falciparum*-related deaths by up to 40% and national bed net programmes are being implemented in a number of sub-Saharan African countries (D'Alessandro et al 1995a). However, it is widely accepted that long-term control of malaria depends upon the development of a safe, cheap and highly immunogenic vaccine.

It has long been known that residents of highly malaria endemic areas acquire protective (but non-sterilizing) immunity to malaria. Young children are susceptible to disease and death but, following infection, parasite prevalence, parasite density and the number of clinical episodes decline progressively. Adults are more or less resistant to the pathologic effects of infection (McGregor 1986). If this process could be mimicked by vaccination, severe malaria and malaria-related deaths could be prevented. Such a vaccine would need to target the intra-erythrocytic stage of the life-cycle, which is responsible for the clinical symptoms and severe pathology of the disease, and would need to induce lifelong immunity which could be boosted by periodic reinfection. The aim of vaccination would be to inhibit merozoite replication or erythrocyte invasion, thereby keeping parasite density below the threshold required to trigger an inflammatory response. An alternative approach, from a public health perspective, is to limit the spread of malaria by targeting the transmission stages of the life-cycle which infect mosquitoes. Finally, a vaccine which effectively targets the infective (sporozoite) stages would completely prevent infection and may also be suitable for travellers from non-endemic countries.

Early Vaccine Studies

Early attempts to produce a malaria vaccine were largely empirical and followed the tried and tested approach of pathogen attenuation—in this case irradiation of sporozoite-infected mosquitoes. Irradiated mosquitoes were allowed to feed on (and infect) non-immune human volunteers who were then challenged with bites from infected, non-irradiated mosquitoes and monitored for signs of infection. Protective immunity was induced but was short lived and species specific (Rieckmann et al 1979). Protected individuals had serum antibodies to the surface-coat protein of the sporozoite, the circumsporozite protein, and it seemed plausible that these antibodies were mediating protection.

Malaria vaccine research was revolutionized in the late 1970s by the development of methods for long term in-vitro culture of *P. falciparum* and by recombinant DNA technology. The gene for the *P. falciparum* circumsporozoite protein was cloned in 1984 and human clinical trials, with a recombinant protein vaccine and a synthetic peptide vaccine, commenced in 1986. Unfortunately, these first generation anti-malaria vaccines were poorly immunogenic and did not confer protection to most vaccinated individuals (Ballou et al 1987; Herrington et al 1987). It was subsequently realized that highly immune individuals living in endemic areas, who had very high titres of anti-sporozoite antibodies, were not actually protected against infection and would periodically be infected by blood-stage parasites (Hoffman et al 1987). At about the same time, it was realized that heavily irradiated sporozoites, which failed to invade hepatocytes, were not able to induce protective immunity. Attention moved from the sporozoite itself to intrahepatic parasites and non-antibody-mediated immune mechanisms were explored.

These early studies were extremely instructive. Firstly, it became clear that although the attenuated vaccine approach might be theoretically possible, it was not feasible to produce parasites on the scale required and the only way forward was through recombinant DNA or synthetic peptide technology. Secondly, the simplistic approach of identifying an antigen on the basis of its recognition by immune serum, genetically engineering its production and injecting it with a standard adjuvant (alum) (Ballou et al 1987) or carrier antigen (tetanus toxoid) (Herrington et al 1987) was probably not going to work. Thirdly, there was a lot that could be learned about immune effector mechanisms in malaria by studying naturally acquired immune responses in malaria-exposed populations.

Correspondence: E. Riley, Institute of Cell, Animal and Population Biology, Ashworth Laboratories, University of Edinburgh, Edinburgh, EH9 3JT, UK. E-Mail: e.riley@ed.ac.uk

More recently, workers have had a much more focussed idea of what they expect a particular malaria vaccine to achieve, what the longterm benefits and potential hazards of vaccine implementation might be, how the vaccine should be formulated and how it can be evaluated.

Requirements for a Malaria Vaccine

The main market for a malaria vaccine will be in developing or newly industrialized countries. The health budgets of such countries are small and already overstretched. A malaria vaccine will need to provide a clear cost benefit—i.e. the cost of implementing a vaccine programme must be recoverable in terms of decreased treatment costs. This means that the vaccine must be cheap to buy and easy to administer. It should be stable at ambient temperatures (which can rise above 40°C in many endemic countries) to avoid the cost of cold storage and the risk of vaccine failure after breaks in the cold-chain. Ideally the vaccine should be highly immunogenic, protecting more than 90% of individuals after a single dose and being boosted by re-exposure in the field. In countries with poor infrastructure and highly mobile populations, vaccine programmes which require multiple injections and frequent boosting will rapidly breakdown. Maximum uptake of the vaccine will be achieved if it can be integrated into the existing WHO-sponsored expanded programme of immunization (EPI) for childhood diseases. Finally, the vaccine must be able to protect against all genotypes of malaria parasites, which means targeting conserved or semi-conserved antigens.

To date, most of the research effort has been put into a vaccine against falciparum malaria—partly because it is the most serious and most widespread of the human malarias but also because the development of in-vitro culture techniques for this parasite has made it much more accessible to laboratory workers. *Plasmodium vivax* is now receiving more attention and, with the benefit of experience gained with *P. falciparum*, research is moving ahead rapidly. There is still considerable debate about the extent of cross-immunity between the two species. In areas where both diseases occur together, there is a tendency to assume that some cross-immunity exists, although much of the data is anecdotal. There are regions of genetic sequence conservation between different *Plasmodium* spp but little evidence for widespread antigenic conservation, although the endotoxin-like molecules produced by rupturing schizonts are immunologically cross-reactive (Bate et al 1992)—which may explain why the clinical symptoms of falciparum malaria appear to be ameliorated in individuals with previous experience of vivax malaria. For the most part, however, it seems that separate vaccines will be required to protect against the two species of malaria.

Evaluation of Vaccine Candidates

Thus far, there are no reliable in-vitro tests which will predict whether an individual is protected against further malaria infection or disease. Response to vaccination can be monitored by sero-conversion or activation of various cellular mechanisms but these parameters do not necessarily correlate with protective immunity. Antibody screening may be of use for confirming vaccine viability and general immunogenicity during the implementation phase of a vaccine programme but may be of little use in monitoring vaccine efficacy during clinical or pre-clinical trials. The most promising surrogate measure of protection against blood-stage parasites seems to be the ability of immune serum to mediate antibody-dependent killing of intra-erythrocytic parasites (Bouharoun-Tayoun et al 1990) but the correlation only holds at a population level and will not predict whether specific individuals are protected. Also, this method is too cumbersome for wide-scale use in the monitoring of vaccine trials.

There are no completely appropriate animal models of human malaria. Immunization and challenge of New World monkeys is useful, although variation in individual monkey susceptibility to *P. falciparum* infection means that several animals need to be used in each experiment to assure a statistically significant result (Anon 1988). In the limited number of cases where human malaria vaccine trials have followed apparently successful monkey experiments, correlation between protection in monkeys and humans has been disappointing and some researchers are now questioning the value of such experiments.

The only certain way to evaluate new malaria vaccines is in clinical trials, which is time consuming and expensive. There are also ethical problems. On the whole, the countries where malaria vaccines are to be tested do not have their own indigenous vaccine development programmes. Health officials in these countries are being asked to make difficult decisions about the relative merits of different vaccine candidates and may be under pressure to cooperate with overseas funding agencies. Fortunately, WHO has undertaken the role of vaccine trials coordinator, acting as an independent scrutineer of preclinical data, defining trial protocols and matching candidate vaccines to appropriate trial sites.

Selection of Immunogens

Malaria parasites are genetically complex. Their genome contains somewhere between 3000 and 4000 genes, compared with an average of 30–40 genes in a relatively complex virus. Malaria parasites are also extremely genetically diverse and have demonstrated the ability to adapt rapidly to adverse circumstances, for example the spread of drug resistance (Walliker 1994). Antigenic polymorphism is the rule rather than the exception for malaria antigens, particularly for antigens on the surface of the parasite or infected host cells which are exposed to the immune system. Anti-malarial immunity is believed to be at least partially strain-specific although definitive epidemiological studies of the relative importance of strain-specific responses are only now being undertaken.

Although some malaria antigens are expressed throughout the life-cycle, each stage of the life-cycle expresses novel antigens. For example, the circumsporozoite protein is expressed on the surface of sporozoites and can be found in early liver-stage parasites and in the mature oocyst. Specific antigens are expressed on liver-stage schizonts which differ from those expressed on intra-erythrocytic schizonts and the sexual stages express another set of surface antigens. These antigens are not immunologically cross-reactive so that immunity raised to one parasite stage will not protect against other stages. Thus a vaccine based on the circumsporozoite protein would not protect against blood-stage parasites and if a single sporozoite successfully matured into a liver schizont, a full blown blood-stage infection could follow. Similarly, a vaccine which reduced the development of asexual stages would not affect sexual-stage parasites—which may lead to selection for highly transmissible strains of parasite which have evolved to very early gametocyte production, as is believed to have occurred after the introduction of mass chemoprophylaxis in Africa, reviewed by Carter & Graves (1988). On the other hand, the formulation of a multi-stage vaccine, simultaneously targeting several different antigens, would allow the various immune responses to act synergistically, increasing the overall efficacy of the vaccine and hindering the spread of vaccine escape mutants.

For an antigen to be targeted by antibody-mediated immune effector mechanisms, it has to be expressed either on the surface of the parasite itself, or on the surface of the infected hepatocyte or erythrocyte. Malaria parasites are intracellular for most of the time, but sporozoites are vulnerable during the infection process, merozoites are extracellular during schizont rupture and reinvasion and gametocytes give rise to extracellular gametes in the midgut of the mosquito, where they are exposed to all the components of the blood meal including antibody, cells and complement (Carter et al 1988). In order to survive within the host cell, the parasite must modify the cell in various ways. This includes the insertion of parasite-derived antigens, such as specific transporter molecules, into the host cell membrane. In the case of *P. falciparum*, specific adhesion molecules are expressed on the surface of the parasitized erythrocyte which allow schizont-infected cells to adhere to the endothelium of post-capillary venules and thus avoid immune clearance in the spleen (Schlichtherle et al 1996). These cell-surface antigens are exposed to the immune system throughout the period of infection of the cell and are thus tempting targets for immune intervention to induce antibodies which inhibit cytoadherence and facilitate immune clearance of parasitized red blood cells.

Cell-mediated effector mechanisms can be triggered by virtually any parasite antigen. Dead parasites are phagocytosed and their constituent proteins expressed on the surface of antigen-presenting cells where they activate T cells. When these T cells subsequently come into contact with dead or dying parasites, or parasite antigens expressed on host cells, they may be directly cytotoxic (cytotoxic T lymphocytes, CTLs) or may induce the production of inflammatory mediators and parasiticidal molecules such as nitric oxide (Long 1993). The only parasite stage which is susceptible to CD8+ CTLs is the intrahepatocytic stage, as human red blood cells do not express class I major histocompatibility complex (MHC) antigens. There has been considerable interest in the possible role of CTLs in anti-malarial immunity ever since these cells were found to confer immunity to malaria in mouse models (Romero et al 1988), however recent evidence throws doubt on the role of direct cellular cytotoxicity as the effector mechanism and it now seems likely that the effects are partly cytokine-mediated.

Another logical approach to vaccine development would be to target molecules which perform vital parasite functions. Such molecules tend to be functionally constrained in their structure and are thus less polymorphic. Potential targets include parasite-specific enzymes (such as those within the folate pathway, which have been inhibited pharmacologically) or molecules involved in the cellular invasion process (Holder

& Blackman 1994). Finally, many of the pathological effects of malaria infection are believed to be mediated by parasite-derived endotoxin-like molecules, phospholipoproteins which may be derived from the glycophosphoinositol anchors attaching proteins to the parasite surface membrane (Schofield & Hackett 1993). The toxins of different malaria species are immunologically cross-reactive and neutralizing antibodies to them inhibit the induction of pro-inflammatory cytokine responses (Bate et al 1992). An anti-toxic vaccine thus has the potential to protect against clinical malaria but would need to be used in conjunction with an anti-merozoite vaccine to limit parasite growth. One disadvantage of this approach is that the toxins tend to induce T-cell-independent immune responses which are of low affinity and short duration (Bate et al 1990)—although this problem could be overcome by coupling the toxin to a protein carrier molecule. More problematic is the likelihood that these complex glycolipoproteins may be very difficult to synthesize.

Identification of potential vaccine targets is only part of the process; selecting which ones to follow up requires additional information. In the early days (1985 or thereabouts), candidate molecules were identified by immunoblotting with immune serum and their genes were cloned by screening expression libraries with the same serum. Some of these antigens are still prime candidates but many others have been exhaustively characterized but finally abandoned because, although they were highly immunogenic, the immune responses to them were not protective. Protective responses can be differentiated from non-protective responses by a variety of means including in-vitro testing of their ability to inhibit parasite growth or infectivity, or by immuno-epidemiological methods, looking for associations between immune responses and clinical immunity in endemic populations. As discussed above, these methods are by no means foolproof, but they do provide some objective criteria by which candidate antigens can be prioritized for further study. The immunological approach to malaria vaccine development has recently been extensively reviewed (Hoffman 1996).

Current Status of Candidate Vaccine Antigens

Pre-erythrocytic stage vaccines

Currently, two sporozoite surface antigens, the circumsporozoite protein and sporozoite surface antigen 2 (SSP2), and a number of liver-stage specific antigens, including liver-stage antigen 1 (LSA1), LSA2 and the sporozoite and liver-stage antigen (SALSA), are being evaluated as potential vaccine antigens. For the sporozoite proteins the main problem appears to be generating a construct which induces very high titre antibodies. Numerous approaches have been tried including expression in vaccinia virus, use of immuno-stimulating complexes (ISCOMS) and multiple antigenic peptides (MAP). More recently DNA vaccines have been explored (Hoffman 1996). Small-scale (Phase 1) human trials have been, and are being, conducted with a variety of immunogens but no large-scale clinical trials have been undertaken.

For the liver-stage antigens, formulations to induce cell-mediated immune mechanisms (CTL- and cytokine-mediated) are being evaluated (Nardin & Nussenzweig 1993). Although there is no direct evidence that CTLs are involved in protective immunity to malaria in humans, cloned CTLs are able to confer protection in murine malaria, and lymphocytes from malaria-immune humans mediate lysis of target cells loaded with sporozoite or liver-stage antigen-derived peptides (Malik et al 1991). Given the diversity of HLA Class I alleles in human populations, defining a peptide vaccine which will induce CTLs in all, or a majority, of potential recipients may prove difficult.

Antigenic polymorphism does not appear to be such a major problem for pre-erythrocytic antigens as for blood-stage antigens. Variation in T-cell epitopes of the circumsporozoite protein has been described (Good et al 1988) but conserved T-cell epitopes have been identified which are recognized in association with most MHC class II alleles (Sinigaglia et al 1988). There are subtle variations in the sequence and number of tetrapeptide repeats which form the immunodominant B-cell epitopes, but these sequence variations do not appear to translate into significant antigenic polymorphism. LSA1 is highly conserved and contains well recognized T- and B-cell epitopes, including epitopes for CTLs (Fidock et al 1994).

Erythrocytic stage vaccines

Approaches to blood-stage vaccine development include induction of antibodies which mediate phagocytosis or cellular cytotoxicity of free merozoites, inhibit ligand-receptor interactions involved in merozoite invasion of erythrocytes or target essential enzymes. Antibody-independent mechanisms include induction of inhibitory cytokines and toxic radicals (Long 1993). Currently, two merozoite surface membrane antigens (merozoite surface protein 1, MSP1, and MSP2) and the apical membrane antigen (AMA-1) are undergoing safety and immunogenicity trials in humans, and efficacy trials in monkeys. Of these, a 19 kDa fragment from the C-terminus of MSP1 ($MSP1_{19}$) induces antibodies which are associated with protective immunity in humans (Riley et al 1992; Egan et al 1995). $MSP1_{19}$ has been expressed as a correctly folded protein in bacterial, yeast, insect (baculovirus) and vaccinia expression systems. The first three of these yielded highly immunogenic proteins but only the yeast and baculovirus products were able to induce protective immunity in monkeys and protection was dependent on the use of Freund's adjuvant (Kumar et al 1995; Chang et al 1996). Phase 1 human trials have begun with the yeast product, using alum as adjuvant, but no results have yet been reported.

The family of genes encoding the parasite-derived erythrocyte membrane proteins (PfEMP1) , which are believed to be involved in parasite cytoadherence and sequestration, have recently been identified (Borst et al 1995), opening up the possibility of exploiting these antigens as vaccines. The antigens appear to be highly immunogenic but they are extremely polymorphic and undergo clonal antigenic variation such that several different antigens are sequentially expressed by a single parasite clone during the course of a single blood-stage infection. From the data collected so far there appears to be very little sequence conservation between different members of the family, making it difficult to conceive how they might form the basis of a strain-independent vaccine. However, the function of PfEMP1 (cytoadherence to a small number of host adhesion molecules) is relatively conserved implying that there is conservation of crucial structures at the three-dimensional level even if there is little in the way of linear sequence homology. Recently described techniques such as random display of peptides on the surface of bacteriophage may be one way of identifying such 3-D structures (Schlichtherle et al 1996).

To date, the only asexual-stage malaria vaccine to have undergone multiple field trials is the synthetic peptide vaccine developed in Colombia by Dr Manuel Patarroyo (Moreno & Patarroyo 1989). The vaccine has been, and still is, the focus of unprecedented controversy (Maurice 1995). SPf66 was developed empirically by immunizing wild-caught *Aotus trivirgatus* monkeys with affinity-purified merozoite-derived proteins and challenging them with *P. falciparum*. Proteins which conferred some degree of immunity were partially sequenced and synthetic peptides derived from these sequences were used to immunize more monkeys. Promising peptides were combined and the most effective combination synthesized as a single hybrid polypeptide which was then polymerized (SPf66). The polymer contains sequences derived from three separate merozoite antigens (including an *N*-terminal sequence of MSP1) linked by a sequence derived from the repetitive B-cell epitope (NANP) of the circumsporozoite protein. Partial protection in some animals was observed in monkey trials (Patarroyo et al 1987) but two independent research teams were unable to reproduce these results (Herrera et al 1990; Ruebush et al 1990). In the first human trial of SPf66, levels of protection similar to those observed in the original monkey trial were obtained (Patarroyo et al 1988); 3 of 5 volunteers resolved a challenge infection without treatment but all volunteers developed clinical symptoms of malaria (fever, headache, nausea). There was no correlation between protection and any measured immunological parameter.

In the course of four combined safety, immunogenicity and efficacy trials in South America between 1988 and 1993, approximately 18 000 people received the SPf66 vaccine (Tanner et al 1995). Although the vaccine seemed safe, and estimates of efficacy varied from 30 to 80%, significant doubts remained. In the first three trials, estimates of efficacy were based on rather small numbers of clinical cases and the trials were either not properly randomized or had inappropriate controls. An independent randomized, double-blind, placebo-controlled trial of SPf66 was conducted in Tanzanian children in 1993. The vaccine had no effect on the incidence of infection or parasite density in asymptomatic infections but 58 cases of clinical malaria were identified in 274 vaccinated children and 88 cases in 312 placebo recipients—giving a risk ratio of 0·72 and an estimated vaccine efficacy of 31% (95% confidence interval, 0–52%) (Alonso et al 1994). A second independent trial in The Gambia (D'Alessandro et al 1995b) showed no protective effect of SPf66 vaccination in children under one year of age (7·1 clinical cases per 1000 child days at risk in the vaccinated group, 7·2 cases per 1000 days at risk in the unvaccinated group). Vaccinated children did, however, have high titres of specific antibody, indicating that they had responded well to the peptide immunogen. No protection against clinical malaria was observed and there were no significant differences between vaccinated and unvaccinated children in terms of parasite prevalence, parasite density or any other measure of malaria-related morbidity. A third independent trial in children in Thailand was similarly disappointing (Nosten et al 1996).

Despite their shortcomings, the first five trials all suggested that vaccinated individuals are at marginally lower risk of clinical malaria than are unvaccinated individuals, but the protective efficacy is exceedingly small – too small to be measured accurately even in large field trials. The Tanzanian trial was restricted to children aged 1 to 5 years but previous studies in the same population have shown that most malaria-attributable morbidity occurs in children under 1 year of age (Smith et al 1995). In contrast, the Gambian trial targeted children aged 6–9 months, precisely the time at which maternal immunity wanes and children become highly susceptible to infection—and the children were not protected. This suggests that the vaccine may be able to boost an existing immune response but is not able to immunise essentially naive individuals. There is no evidence so far that the vaccine prevents severe disease or death; mortality trials are necessarily very large and it is regarded as unethical to proceed with such a trial unless there is convincing evidence of protection against infection or clinical disease. The SPf66 vaccine is currently being redesigned and new peptide constructs are being evaluated.

Transmission blocking vaccines

The next malaria vaccine to reach full-scale clinical trials is likely to be directed against transmission stages (Kaslow et al 1992). A recombinant, yeast-derived polypeptide representing a zygote-specific surface antigen (Pfs25) induces transmission blocking antibodies which pass into the mosquito midgut, as part of the blood meal, and inactivate the developing ookinete. Human safety and immunogenicity trials of Pfs25 have been completed and preparations are underway for field-based efficacy trials. One disadvantage of Pfs25 as a vaccine antigen is that this protein is not expressed by parasite stages within the human host. Thus, a vaccine-induced immune response will not be boosted by natural reinfection. On the other hand, Pfs25 has a major advantage over other transmission-blocking vaccine candidates in that it has a relatively simple secondary and tertiary structure, allowing its expression as a conformationally correct protein which induces antibodies which bind to the native antigen on the parasite surface. In contrast, the two major surface antigens of gametocytes and gametes (Pfs230 and Pfs48/45), which are both targets of transmission-blocking antibodies, have a complex disulphide-bonded secondary structure which is essential for antibody recognition (Carter et al 1995). It has not yet been possible to express these two antigens in the appropriate conformation for recognition by transmission-blocking monoclonal antibodies or for use in immunization studies. Novel expression strategies may need to be exploited—for example, phage display—to recreate these complex epitopes.

Epidemiological Consequences of Malaria Vaccination

There are several possible outcomes of a successful malaria vaccine programme. Significant reduction of malaria transmission, morbidity and mortality would be considered a major achievement, but there are potential hazards.

Firstly, in endemic areas, the impact of malaria is greatly ameliorated by a high degree of naturally acquired immunity in the population, which is maintained by periodic subclinical infection. Stable endemic malaria is generally less of an acute health-care problem than is unstable epidemic malaria (although the chronic effects of persistent or repeated infec-

tions are frequently underestimated). Significant reduction of malaria transmission after introduction of a vaccine will reduce this natural boosting of immunity and delay the development of naturally acquired immunity in individuals who have not been vaccinated or who have not responded to vaccination. If the vaccine programme fails, and malaria transmission increases, these individuals are vulnerable to infection and are likely to develop symptoms at the severe end of the spectrum of clinical malaria. Importantly, a vaccine which is only partially protective but nevertheless reduces malaria transmission, could transform a stable situation into an epidemic one with a consequent increase in morbidity and mortality. Thus, vaccine programmes need to be integrated into a wider programme of malaria control and vaccines must be evaluated in comparison with and in conjunction with, alternative control measures, such as insecticide-impregnated bed nets.

Secondly, as discussed above, malaria parasites are genetically diverse with the capacity to evolve rapidly in response to a changing environment. The development of vaccine-resistant mutants is to be expected, particularly if the vaccine is based on a single antigenic peptide. In the long term we need to consider multivalent vaccines, targeting different stages of the parasite life-cycle and, preferably, including a transmission-blocking component.

The Future for Malaria Vaccines

In the 1970s and 1980s, numerous pharmaceutical companies, government-sponsored research agencies and international development organizations were investing in malaria vaccine programmes. Rapid progress in the sporozoite vaccine programme held out the prospect of a cheap synthetic vaccine with wide-scale applicability and large profits. However, it is already ten years since the results of the first clinical trials were published and there is still no firm evidence that a protective vaccine is in sight. Lack of definitive progress within the time frame originally envisaged has already led to a reduction in funding by most organizations and some have pulled out altogether. Most of the pharmaceutical companies are now just keeping a close eye on progress within the academic research community rather than investing directly in research and development.

The most successful vaccine programmes have been those where academic research programmes have had long-term financial support for both field-based and laboratory-based research coupled with access to industrial product development. The WHO continues to play a major role in motivating and coordinating the various research programmes, but has little in the way of financial resources to drive the process forward. These financial and political issues will need to be resolved if we are to stand a realistic chance of implementing a vaccine programme in the next 10 or even 20 years.

On the positive side, the last 15 years of intensive effort have paved the way for more rapid progress in the near future. Apart from the antigens highlighted here, there are numerous others which have been identified as potential vaccine candidates (e.g. SERA, EBA-175, RAP1, RAP2). Some of these are now being characterized while others have been shelved due to lack of resources. Several research teams have gained considerable expertise in conducting malaria vaccine trials and more precise definitions of clinical disease have been obtained using data collected during the recent African SPf66 trials (Smith et al 1994). The methodology for conducting multi-centre trials is much more sophisticated than it was 5 years ago and the next generation of trials should be quicker to get off the ground and easier to compare.

References

Alonso, P. L., Smith, T., Armstrong Schellenberg, J. R. M., Masanja, H., Mwankusye, S., Urassa, H., Bastos de Azvedo, I., Chongela, J., Kobero, S., Menendez, C., Hurt, N., Thomas, M. C., Lyimo, E., Weiss, N. A., Hayes, R., Kitua, A. Y., Lopez, M. C., Kilama, W. L., Teuscher, T., Tanner, M. (1994) Randomised trial of efficacy of Spf66 vaccine against Plasmodium falciparum malaria in children in southern Tanzania. Lancet 344: 1175–1181

Anon (1988) Role of non-human primates in malaria vaccine development: memorandum from a WHO meeting. Bull. WHO 66: 719–728

Ballou, W. R., Hoffman, S. L., Sherwood, J. A., Hollingdale M. R., Neva, F. A., Hockmeyer, W. A., Gordon, D. M., Schneider, I., Wirtz, R. A., Young, J. F., Wasserman, G. F., Reeve, P., Diggs, C. L., Chulay, J. D. (1987) Safety and efficacy of a recombinant Plasmodium falciparum sporozoite vaccine. Lancet I: 1277–1281

Bate, C. A. W., Taverne, J., Davé, A., Playfair, J. H. L. (1990) Malaria exoantigens induce T-independent antibody that blocks their ability to induce TNF. Immunol. 70: 315–320

Bate, C. A. W., Taverne, J., Bootsma, H. J., Mason, R. C. S., Skalko, N., Gregoriadis, G., Playfair, J. H. L. (1992) Antibodies against phosphatidylinositol and inositol monophosphate specifically inhibit tmour necrosis factor induction by malaria exoantigens. Immunol. 76: 35–41

Borst, P., Bitter, W., McCulloch, R., Van Leeuwen, F., Rudenko, G. (1995) Antigenic variation in malaria. Cell 82: 1–4

Bouharoun-Tayoun, H., Attanath, P., Sabcharoen, A., Chongsuphajaisiddhi, T., Druilhe, P. (1990) Antibodies that protect humans against Plasmodium falciparum blood stages do not on their own inhibit parasite growth and invasion in vitro but act in co-operation with monocytes. J. Exp. Med. 172: 1633–1641

Carter, R., Graves, P. M. (1988) Gametocytes. In: Wernsdorfer, W. H., McGregor, I. (eds) Malaria: Principles and Practice of Malariology. Churchill Livingstone, Edinburgh, pp 253–306

Carter, R., Kumar, N., Quakyi, I. A., Good, M., Mendis, K., Graves, P., Miller, L. (1988) Immunity to sexual stages of malaria parasites. Prog. Allergy 41: 193–214

Carter, R., Coulson, A., Bhatti, S., Taylor, B. J., Elliott, J. F. (1995) Predictedy disulfide-bonded structures for three uniquely related proteins of Plasmodium falciparum, Pfs230, Pfs48/45 and Pf12. Mol. Biochem. Parasitol. 71: 203–210

Chang, S. P., Case, S. E., Gosnell, W. L., Hashimoto, A., Kramer, K. J., Tam, L. Q., Hashiro, C. Q., Nikaido, C. M., Gibson, H. L., Lee-Ng, C. T., Barr, P. J., Yokota, B. T., Hui, G. S. N. (1996) A recombinant baculovirus 42-kilodalton C-terminal fragment of Plasmodium falciparum merozoite surface protein 1 protects Aotus monkeys against malaria. Infect. Immun. 64: 253–261

D'Alessandro, U., Olaleye, B., McGuire, W., Langerock, P., Bennett, S., Aikins, M. K., Thomson, M. C., Cham, M. K., Greenwood, B. M. (1995a) Mortality and morbidity from malaria in Gambian children after introduction of an impregnated bednet programme. Lancet 345:479–483

D'Alessandro, U., Leach, A., Drakeley, C. J., Bennett, S., Olaleye, B., Fegan, G. W., Juwara, M., Langerock, P., George, M. O., Targett, G. A. T., Greenwood, B. M. (1995b) Efficacy trial of malaria vaccine SPf66 in Gambian infants. Lancet 346: 462–467

Egan, A. F., Morris, J., Barnish, G., Allen, S., Greenwood, B. M., Kaslow, D. C., Holder, A. A., Riley, E. M. (1995) Clinical immunity to Plasmodium falciparum malaria is associated with serum antibodies to the 19kDa C-terminal fragment of the merozoite surface antigen, PfMSP1. J. Infect. Dis. 173: 765–769

Fidock, D. A., Gras-Masse, H., Lepers, J., Brahimi, K., Benmohammed, L., Mellouk, S., Guerin-Marchand, C., Londono, A., Raharimalala, L., Meis, J. F. G. M., Langsley, G., Roussilhon, C., Tartar, A., Druilhe, P. (1994) Plasmodium falciparum liver stage antigen-1 is well conserved and contains potent B and T cell determinants. J. Immunol. 153: 190–204

Good, M. F., Pombo, D., Quakyi, I. A., Riley, E. M., Houghten, R. A., Menon, A., Alling, D. W., Berzofsky, J. A., Miller, L. H. (1988) Human T cell recognition of the circumsporozoite protein of Plasmodium falciparum. Immunodominant T cell domains map to the polymorphic regions of the molecule. Proc. Natl Acad. Sci. USA 85: 1199–1203

Herrera, S., Herrera, M., Corredor, A., Rosero, F., Clavijo, C., Guerrero, R. (1990) Failure of a synthetic vaccine to protect Aotus lemurinus against asexual blood stages of Plasmodium falciparum. Am. J. Trop. Med. Hyg. 47: 682–690

Herrington, D. A., Clyde, D. F., Losonsky, G., Cortesia, M., Murphy, J. R., Davis, J., Baqar, S., Felix, A. M., Heimer, E. P., Gillessen, D., Nardin, E., Nussenzweig, R. S., Hollingdale, M. R., Levine, M. M. (1987). Safety and immunogenicity in man of a synthetic peptide malaria vaccine against Plasmodium falciparum sporozoites. Nature 328: 257–259

Hoffman S. L. (ed.) (1996) Malaria Vaccine Development: A Multi-immune Response Approach. American Society for Microbiology Press, Washington DC

Hoffman, S. L., Oster, C N., Plowe, C. V., Woollett, G. R., Beier, J. C., Chulay, J. D., Wirtz, R. A., Hollingdale, M. R., Mugambi, M. (1987) Naturally acquired antibodies to sporozoites do not prevent malaria: vaccine development implications. Science 237: 639–642

Holder, A. A., Blackman, M. J. (1994) What is the function of MSP-1 on the malaria merozoite? Parasitol. Today 10: 182–184

Kaslow, D. C., Bathurst, I. C., Barr, P. J. (1992) Malaria transmission-blocking vaccines. Trends Biotech. 10: 388–391

Kumar, S., Yadava, A., Keister, D. B., Tian, J. H., Ohl, M., Perdue-Greenfield, K. A., Miller, L. H., Kaslow, D. C. (1995) Immunogenicity and in vivo efficacy of recombinant Plasmodium falciparum merozoite surface protein-1 in Aotus monkeys. Mol. Med. 1: 325–332

Long, C. A. (1993) Immunity to blood stages of malaria. Curr. Opinion Immunol. 5: 548–556

Malik, A., Egan, J. E., Houghten, R., Sadoff, J. C., Hoffman, S. L. (1991) Human cytotoxic T lymphocytes against the Plasmodium falciparum circumsporozoite protein. Proc. Natl Acad. Sci. USA 88: 3300–3304

Maurice, J. (1995) Malaria vaccine raises a dilemma. Science 267: 320–323

McGregor, I. A. (1986) The development and maintenance of immunity to malaria in highly endemic areas. Clin. Trop. Med. Commun. Dis. 1: 29–53

Moreno, A., Patarroyo, M. E. (1989) Development of an asexual blood stage malaria vaccine. Blood 74: 537–546

Nardin, E. H., Nussenzweig, R. S. (1993) T cell responses to pre-erythrocytic stages of malaria: role in protection and vaccine development against pre-erythrocytic stages. Annu. Rev. Immunol. 11: 687–727

Nosten, F., Luxemburger, C., Kyle, D. E., Ballou, W. R., Wittes, J., Wah, P., Chongsuphajaisiddhi, T., Gordon, D. M., White, N. J., Sadoff, J., Heppner, D. G. (1996) Randomised double-blind placebo-controlled trial of Spf66 malaria vaccine in children in north-western Thailand. Lancet 348: 701–708

Patarroyo, M. E., Romero, P., Torres, M. L., Clavijo, P., Moreno, A., Martinez, A., Rodriguez, R., Guzman, F., Cabezas, E. (1987) Induction of protective immunity against experimental infection with malaria using synthetic peptides. Nature 328: 629–632

Patarroyo, M. E., Amador, R., Clavijo, P., Moreno, A., Guzman, F., Romero, P., Tascon, R., Franco, A., Murillo, L. A., Ponton, G., Trujillo, G. (1988) A synthetic vaccine protects humans against challenge with asexual blood stages of Plasmodium falciparum malaria. Nature 332: 158–161

Rieckmann, K. H., Beaudoin, R. L., Cassells, J. S., Sell, K. W. (1979) Use of attenuated sporozoites in the immunization of human volunteers against falciparum malaria. Bull. World Health Organization 57 (Suppl.): 261–265

Riley, E. M., Allen, S. J., Wheeler, J., Blackman, M. J., Bennett, S., Takacs, B., Shönfeld, H., Holder, A. A., Greenwood, B. M. (1992) Naturally acquired cellular and humoral immune responses to the major merozoite surface antigen of Plasmodium falciparum are associated with reduced malaria morbidity. Parasite Immunol. 14: 321–338

Romero, P., Maryanski,J. L., Corradin, G. P., Nussenzweig, R. S., Nussenzweig, V., Zavala, F. (1988) Cloned cytotoxic T cells recognize an epitope in the circumsporozoite protein and protect against malaria. Nature 341: 323–326

Ruebush, T. K., Campbell, G. H., Moreno, A., Patarroyo, M. E., Collins, W. E. (1990) Immunization of owl monkeys with a combination of *Plasmodium falciparum* asexual blood stage synthetic peptide antigens. Am. J. Trop. Med. Hyg. 43: 355–366

Schlichtherle, I. M., Treutiger, C. J., Fernandez, V., Carlson, J., Wahlgren, M. (1996) Molecular aspects of severe malaria. Parasitol. Today 12: 329–332

Schofield, L., Hackett, F. (1993) Signal transduction in host cells by a glycophosphatidylinositol toxin of malaria parasites. J. Exp. Med. 177: 145–153

Sinigaglia, F., Guttinger, M., Kilgus, J., Doran, D. M., Matile, H., Etlinger, H., Trzeciak, A., Gillessen, D., Pink, J. R. L. (1988) A malaria T-cell epitope recognised with most mouse and human MHC class II antigens. Nature 336: 778–780

Smith, T., Schellenberg, J. A., Hayes, R. J. (1994) Attributable fraction estimates and case definitions for malaria in endemic areas. Stat. Med. 13: 2345–2358

Smith, T., Hurt, N., Teuscher, T., Tanner, M. (1995). Is fever a good sign for clinical malaria in surveys of endemic communities? Am. J. Trop. Med. Hyg. 52: 306–310

Tanner, M., Teuscher, T., Alonso, P. L. (1995) Spf66 – The first malaria vaccine. Parasitol. Today 11: 10–13

Walliker, D. (1994) The role of molecular genetics in field studies on malaria parasites. Int. J. Parasitol. 24: 799–808

J. Pharm. Pharmacol. 1997, 49 (Suppl. 2): 29–33

New Targets for Antimalarial Drug Discovery

P. OLLIARO AND D. WIRTH*

UNDP/World Bank/WHO Special Programme for Research and Training in Tropical Diseases (TDR), Geneva, Switzerland, and *Harvard School of Tropical Public Health, Boston MA, USA

The emergence and spread of parasite resistance to in-use antimalarials urges for novel compounds to be discovered and developed. Current research focusses on targets of the growing and dividing parasite (ring, trophozoite, schizont) in the red blood cell (RBC). Those processes are metabolically intense and contain essential targets for parasite survival. Mature intra-erythrocytic stages are also responsible for the severe manifestation of falciparum malaria. *Plasmodium falciparum* is the main focus because it is the most common of the four *Plasmodium* species which commonly infect humans, causes a potentially life-threatening infection, and is also the species which shows the highest levels of resistance to various antimalarials.

Research Priorities for Antimalarial Drug Discovery

The Steering Committee on Drugs for Malaria (CHEMAL) of the World Health Organization's (WHO) Special Programme for Research and Training in Tropical Diseases (TDR) is committed to a concerted, systematic effort for antimalarial drug development involving: identification of chemotherapeutic targets; development of methods to expedite experimentation (gene cloning, protein expression, high throughput assay development, determination of specificity); identification of leads, optimization of inhibitors; and the subsequent pre-clinical and clinical development work. This is being approached by combining efforts of university and government researchers in the discovery area and then developing potential drugs through contracts and industrial partners. Special emphasis is being put on establishing Research & Development (R & D) capability in the developing world. Target generation and validation is one of CHEMAL's top priorities. Emphasis is being put on validating selected targets, and on obtaining and testing compounds for specific inhibition of the target and for activity against the whole parasite. There is a recognized need for more information on the basic metabolic and biochemical processes of the malaria parasite in order to identify the targets for the future. CHEMAL has focussed on targets generation and validation and is now concentrating on those that have been validated, but has also come to recognize that not many of those investigated will ever become validated targets and will generate effective and safe compounds. Hence the need for the discovery and characterization of unique drug targets with specific consideration for the targets which differentiate host and parasite enzymes, as well as for the molecular modelling of host and parasite enzymes. The putative target must be an essential feature of the parasite life-cycle, be parasite-specific (e.g., targets in the digestive vacuole: proteinases, haem polymerization; mitochondrion/plastid) and/or

Correspondence: P. Olliaro, World Health Organization, Avenue Appia, 1211 Geneva 27, Switzerland.

show differential sensitivity from any analogous process in the host (e.g., dihydrofolate reductase, signal transduction). It is also important that some known specific inhibitors exist as a starting point for synthesis (e.g., dihydrofolate reductase, proteinase inhibitors).

Status of New Targets for Antimalarial Drug Development

Through a combination of research in academic centres, governmental research organizations and drug discovery efforts in pharmaceutical companies, a number of new potential target pathways have been identified and these are summarized in the Table 1 and below. Efforts to develop lead compounds for these putative targets are a priority of CHEMAL.

The Plasmodium digestive vacuole

The digestive vacuole (an acidic lysosome-like organelle) contains key processes including haemoglobin metabolism and detoxification and also drug accumulation, which represent potential chemotherapeutic targets (Olliaro & Goldberg 1995). Haemoglobin is ingested by the malaria parasite and processed in the vacuole, where it is digested, and haem, the eventual by-product, is detoxified (Goldberg et al 1990).

Haemoglobin digestion: proteinases inhibitors. To date, three enzymes have been shown to account for the majority of haemoglobin degradation: two aspartic proteases (aspartic haemoglobinase I and II, or plasmodium aspartic proteinase I and II, systematically renamed Plasmepsin I and II by the IUB Nomenclature Committee) have been isolated (Gluzman et al 1994) and the respective genes cloned and sequenced (Dame et al 1994; Francis at al 1994); and one cystein protease (falcipain) (Rosenthal et al 1988, 1991; Rosenthal & Nelson 1992). The aspartic and cystein proteinases are analogous to human cathepsin D and L, respectively. Proteinase inhibition is identified as a priority project for multiple reasons, although the demonstration of the ultimate therapeutic potential of drugs targeted against malaria proteinases remains to be determined. The genes are cloned and sequenced and recombinant proteins expressed in active form and automated assays for proteinase inhibition are available also for homologous human enzymes. Significant differences in amino acid sequence from the corresponding host enzymes and preliminary data with inhibitors substantiate the validity of proteinases as targets. There is potential for piggy-backing on compound libraries from other indications: proteinases are key enzymes in a variety of infectious and non-infectious diseases ranging from HIV to hypertension and arthritis, and inhibitors are being actively sought and developed (Olliaro et al 1996).

Table 1. Potential target pathways for antimalarial therapy.

Target	Validated	Expressed active form	Assay for automation	Mammal target
Haemozoin polymerization	?	NA	Y	?
Plasmepsin I	by inhibition	Y	Y	Y
Plasmepsin II	?	Y	Y	Y
Falcipain	by inhibition	Y	Y	Y
pmfmdr-1	?	Y	Y	Y
DHFR-TS	Y	Y	Y	Y
PPPK-DHPS	Y	Y	Y	Y
HGPRT	Y	Y	N	Y
Ca-dependent protein kinase C	by inhibition	?	N	Y
Ribonucleotide reductase	by inhibition	Y	N	Y
DNA polymerase alpha	?	N	N	Y
Organelle RNA polymerase	N	N	N	Y
Tubulin	N	N	N	Y
Superoxide dismutase	N	?	N	Y
Phosphocholine cytidylyl transferase	?	N	N	?

DHFR-TS, dihydrofolate reductase and thymidylate synthase; PPPK-DHPS, dihydropterate synthase and 2-amino-4-hydroxy-6-hydroxymethyldihydropteridine pyrophosphokinease; HGPRT, hypoxanthine-guanine phosphoribosyl transferase.
? = uncertain; NA = not availabe; Y = yes; N = no.

Haem detoxification. The parasite has developed means to polymerize the otherwise toxic free haem resulting from haemoglobin proteolysis. Haem polymerization is targeted by antimalarial drugs of the 4-aminoquinoline and arylamino-alcohol families, although the process has not been entirely elucidated yet. A haem polymerase activity was initially described (Chou & Fitch 1992; Slater & Cerami 1992), but subsequent studies have revealed that haem can polymerize non-enzymatically under conditions physico-chemically similar to those of the digestive vacuole (Egan et al 1994; Dorn et al 1995) and this may be initiated by histidine-rich proteins (HRP) (Sullivan et al 1996a). Recent experimental data support the hypothesis that quinoline-haem complexes terminate haem chain extension (Sullivan et al 1996b). The continued interest in haem polymerization, although it is not yet completely validated as a target, stems from various factors: it is an essential feature of the parasite life-cycle and there are no alternative biochemical pathways which circumvent the target; it is unique to the parasite; it is a stable target as resistance to quinoline drugs occurs via different mechanisms; and an assay is now available for screening compounds (Ridley 1997).

Oxidative stress, free radicals and artemisinin-type compounds. *P. falciparum* is eminently susceptible to oxidative stress (Clark et al 1989) and needs to rely on the host to combat it (Fairfield et al 1983). Free radicals are commonly generated in the RBC by the oxidation of haemoglobin to methaemoglobin and presumably also in the digestive vacuole when Fe^{2+} is oxidized to Fe^{3+} in the presence of molecular oxygen. Superoxide radicals (whether they diffuse from the RBC through anionic channels or are produced locally) are converted to hydrogen peroxide by superoxide dismutase (SOD).

Artemisinin-derived intermediates were shown to act as alkylating agents, forming covalent adducts with human serum albumin, haemin and the RBC membrane (Yang et al 1993; Asawamahasakda et al 1994a; Hong et al 1994). The endoperoxide bridge appears essential for antimalarial activity, the bridge-lacking deoxyarteether being found inactive as such

adducts can not be formed (Brossi et al 1988; Asawamahasakda et al 1994b). It has been suggested that haem catalyses the reductive decomposition of the endoperoxide group into a free radical (Meshnick et al 1993; Meshnick 1994) and other electrophilic intermediates (Posner & Oh 1992). This hypothesis is supported by the findings that free radical scavengers antagonize activity (Krungkrai & Yuthavong 1987) but the specific reactions involving free radicals have not been defined so far.

More work is underway to generate both more stable derivatives of artemisinin itself, and totally synthetic trioxanes and tetroxanes. For the former, attention is generally focussing on derivatives which will have slower metabolic breakdown and bypass generation of the dihydro metabolite of artemisinin (the major metabolite of the currently used artemisinin derivatives). Evidence that these derivatives may be less neurotoxic (a prime worry about all standard artemisinin derivatives) is emerging. Other derivatives have enhanced activities in-vitro against both chloroquine-resistant and -sensitive strains of *P. falciparum*. Developments in the synthetic trioxane and tetroxane area are exciting (Posner et al 1994, 1996). Synthetic trioxanes have been prepared which have in-vitro activities ranging from equal to that of artemisinin to several thousand times greater than artemisinin. Also important from drug production and regulatory viewpoints, candidate compounds can be prepared easily, in either an enantiomerically pure or achiral form. These criteria also apply to tetroxanes, which are very easily prepared in a minimum number of steps from cheap, accessible starting compounds.

Drug transport. Another potential target in the food vacuole are transport mechanisms. There is mounting evidence that drug transport plays a major role in mediating drug resistance. One such transporter has been identified in *P. falciparum*, the pfmdr1 gene (Volkman et al 1993), and this gene has been implicated in mefloquine resistance and cross-resistance to halofantrin (Wilson et al 1993). Reversal of resistance has been observed by compounds which are known to inhibit mdr function in other systems such as penfluridol, verapamil and desipramine (Bitonti et al 1988; Kyle et al 1993; Oduola et al 1993). This has lead to the proposal that such reversers could be used in combination with antimalarial drugs to treat drug-resistant infections. This strategy is complicated by the potential interaction of these reversal drugs with the human homologue, the P-glycoprotein, and therefore reversal drugs must be tested on both the parasite and human homologue in order to identify compounds with differential specificity.

Nucleic acids

Nucleic acid metabolism of *Plasmodium* (Hassan & Coombes 1988) differs significantly from the corresponding human pathways. The malaria parasite is unable to synthesize purine de novo and must rely on the host erythrocyte for its main source of purine precursors during its intra-erythrocytic growth (Scheibel & Sherman 1988). Conversely, whilst humans are able both to synthesize and to salvage pyrimidine nucleotides, the intra-erythrocytic malaria parasites can only synthesize pyrimidine nucleotides de-novo, being unable to salvage either pyrimidine bases or nucleosides. The de novo synthesis of pyrimidines also involves para-aminobenzoic acid (PABA) and folate cofactors. In contrast to mammalian cells, malaria parasites are unable to salvage exogenous folates and synthesize these cofactors de novo.

Purine metabolism; hypoxanthine. Although adenosine triphosphate (ATP) is the predominant purine present in human erythrocytes, there is considerable evidence that hypoxanthine, formed during the ATP catabolism, is the immediate purine precursor utilized by the parasite and that the parasite-specific enzymes for hypoxanthine salvage exist. Hypoxanthine salvage rather than adenosine salvage is therefore a potential target for new drug development. Among the various enzymes involved in the hypoxanthine salvage, hypoxanthine-guanine phosphoribosyl transferase (HGPRT), is probably the most promising as a potential chemotherapeutic target since the relevant gene has been cloned and expressed (Vasanthakumar et al 1990) and a mammalian enzyme is available for testing for specificity. However, the yield of both the native and the recombinant enzyme is low and an assay for automation is not yet available.

Pyrimidine metabolism and electron transport. At least four enzymes needed for the conversion of carbamyl phosphate to thymidylate (i.e., dihydroorotate dehydrogenase, orotate phosphoribosyltransferase and orotidine 5′-phosphate decarboxylase) differ from the host enzymes by comprising bifunctional complexes (Gero et al 1981; Rathod & Reyes 1983; Krungkraiet al 1990). A novel naphthoquinone antimalarial, atovaquone, is now available in fixed combination with proguanil. Atovaquone has no cross-resistance with known antimalarials. Although it inhibits parasite dihydroorotate dihydrogenase, the primary target appears to be blockade of pyrimidine synthesis by the inhibition of the respiratory chain of malarial mitochondria at complex III (Hudson 1993). Selectivity and specificity of the target is attributed to different lipophilicity and possibly to different amino acid sequence at the binding site of the protozoan ubiquinone compared to that of mammalian cells.

Other inhibitors of this pathway are being sought. For example, dihydroorotase (DHOase), which catalyses the reaction carbamyl phosphate to dihydroorotate, has been purified and various inhibitors have been synthesized and tested (Krungkrai et al 1992; Seymour et al 1994).

Folate metabolism. Some of the most widely used antimalarials inhibit folate metabolism: sulphonamides and sulphones, which prevent the formation of dihydropterate, are usually combined with pyrimethamine, a dihydrofolate reductase inhibitor. Unlike in mammalian cells, PPPK-DHPS (dihydropterate synthase; and 2-amino-4-hydroxy-6-hydroxymethyldihydropteridine pyrophosphokinase) and DHFR-TS (dihydrofolate reductase and thymidylate synthase) exist in malaria parasites as bifunctional enzymes (Ivanetich & Santi 1990). The genes for DHFR and DHPS are now sequenced and the enzymes expressed in their active form. DHFR mutants are also available. The test can be formatted for high-throughput screening against the human enzymes and there are massive libraries of compounds to test. It is not clear, though, if this can lead to new effective antimalarials. Resistance occurs due to one gene mutation (Hyde 1989; Foote et al 1990; Peterson et al 1990), hence compounds are prone to resistance and are also likely to have a short lifespan. Other enzymes that constitute possible chemotherapeutic targets are serine hydroxymethyltransferase (SHMT) (Rueenwongsa et al 1989), methylene tetrahydrofolate reductase (MTHFR) and methionine synthase (MS) (Asawamahasakda & Yuthavong 1993).

Phospholipid metabolism

Drug discovery and development often ensue from long-term strategic research projects even in the absence of precisely identified targets. One such example is a new family of inhibitors of *Plasmodium* phospholipid metabolism. Intra-erythrocytic stage parasites require large amounts of phospholipid (PL), which is synthesized from plasmatic free fatty acids and polar heads. An accessible target in this pathway is the choline transporter, which provides the intracellular parasite with choline, a precursor required for synthesis of phosphatidylcholine (PC), the major parasite PL. A synthesis effort has produced several hundred molecules with significant structure-activity work. First-generation compounds contained a quaternary ammonium for high antimalarial activity but had availability problems. Newer bioisosters of quaternary ammonium revealed improved absorption and less toxicity (H. Vial, personal communication). In-vitro, the compounds possess high antimalarial activity against chloroquine-sensitive and -resistant *P. falciparum* in the lower nanomolar range, with no cross-resistance with known antimalarials. Selected compounds are also highly potent in-vivo in the *Aotus* monkey model. Predevelopment work is underway on selected leads.

Other pathways

Ongoing research is pointing at a variety of putative chemotherapeutic targets which still await confirmation or have not yet produced significant leads. Some seem more promising than others, namely protein kinase C (Zhao et al 1993), organelle RNA polymerase (Wilson al 1991; Geary & Jensen 1983; Strath et al 1993), ribonucleotide reductase and DNA polymerase alpha. These are targets of known drugs both in humans and in other microbial agents and thus have the potential as targets in the parasite system. Emphasis on target validation is critical at this point.

Perspective

While there are several potential targets for chemotherapeutic intervention which have been identified and are in various stages of target validation or lead identification and optimization, experience in other systems has demonstrated that only a limited number of such leads ever reach even the early stages of drug development. Thus, there is a continuing need for target identification in *Plasmodium*, as there is in other microbial systems. A novel approach to target identification has been initiated through the Malaria Genome Sequencing Project in which the goal will be to determine the complete sequence of *P. falciparum* genome. Advances in sequencing technology have now made such an approach feasible. The complete sequence of several bacterial pathogens has now been completed as has the complete sequence of *Sacchromyces cervisae*. Through a comparison of the sequences of microbial genomes, common essential target enzymes will be identified, as will elements unique to each organism. It is too early to evaluate this approach, however pharmaceutical companies are making major investments in the sequencing of several bacterial pathogens and thus such an investment by the public and philanthropic sectors in *P. falciparum* is timely and appropriate.

Acknowledgements
The authors wish to acknowledge the contribution of current and previous members of CHEMAL, which has lead to the present work plan.

References

Asawamahasakda, V., Yuthavong, Y. (1993) The methionine synthesis cycle and salvage of methyltetrahydrofolate from host red cells in the malaria parasite (*Plasmodium falciparum*). Parasitology 107: 1–10

Asawamahasakda, W., Benakis, A., Meshnick, S. R. (1994a) The interaction of artemisinin with red cell membranes. J. Lab. Clin. Med. 1994 123: 757–762

Asawamahasakda, W., Ittarat, I., Pu, Y. M., Ziffer, H., Meshnick, S. R. (1994b) Reaction of antimalarial endoperoxides with specific parasite proteins. Antimicrob. Agents Chemother. 38: 1854–1858

Bitonti, A. J., Sioerdsma, A., McCann, P. P., Kyle, D. E., Oduola, A. M. J., Rossan, R. N., Milhous, W. K., Davidson, D. E. (1988) Reversal of chloroquine resistance in malaria parasite *Plasmodium falciparum* by desipramine. Science 242: 1301–1303

Brossi, A., Venugopaplan, B., Gerpe, L. D., Yeh, H. J. C., Flippen-Anderson, J. L., Luo, X. D., Milhous, W., Peters, W. (1988) Arteether, a new antimalarial drug: synthesis and antimalarial properties. J. Med. Chem. 31: 645–650

Chou, A. C., Fitch, C. D. (1992) Control of heme polymerase by chloroquine and other quinoline derivatives. Biochem. Biophys. Res. Commun. 195: 422–427

Clark, I. A., Chaudhri, G., Cowden, W. B. (1989) Some roles of free radicals in malaria. Free Radic. Biol. Med. 6: 315–321

Dame, J. B., Reddy, G. R., Yowell, C. A., Dunn, B. M., Kay, J., Berry, C. (1994) Sequence, expression and modeled structure of an aspartic proteinase from the human malaria parasite *Plasmodium falciparum*. Mol. Biochem. Parasitol. 64: 177–190

Dorn, A., Stoffel, R., Matile, H., Bubendorf, A., Ridley, R. (1995) Malarial haemozoin/beta-haematin supports haem polymerization in the absence of protein. Nature 374: 269–271

Egan, T. J., Ross, D. C., Adams, P. A. (1994) Quinoline anti-malarial drugs inhibit spontaneous formation of beta-haematin (malaria pigment). FEBS Lett. 352: 54–57

Fairfield, A. S., Meshnick, S. R., Eaton, J. W. (1983) Malaria parasites adopt host cell superoxide dismutase. Science 221: 764–766

Foote, S. J., Galatis, D., Cowman, A. F.(1990) Amino acids in the dihydrofolate reductase-thymidylate synthase gene of *Plasmodium falciparum* involved in cycloguanil resistance differ from those involved in pyrimethamine resistance. Proc. Natl Acad. Sci. USA 87: 3014–3017

Francis, S. E., Gluzman, I. Y., Oksman, A., Knickerbocker, A., Mueller, R., Bryant, M. L., Sherman, D. R., Russel, D. G., Goldberg, D. E. (1994) Molecular characterization and inhibition of a *Plasmodium falciparum* aspartic hemoglobinase. EMBO J. 13: 306–317

Geary, T. G., Jensen, J. B. (1983) Effects of antibiotics on *Plasmodium falciparum* in vitro. Am. J. Trop. Med. Hyg. 32: 221–225

Gero, A. M., Tetley, K., Coombes, G. H., Phillips, R. S. (1981) Dihydroorotate dehydrogenase, orotate phosphoribosyltransferase and orotidine 5′-phosphate decarboxylase in *Plasmodium falciparum*. Trans. R. Soc. Trop. Med. 75: 719–720

Gluzman, I. Y., Francis, S. E., Oksman, A., Smith, C., Duffin, K., Goldberg, D. G. (1994) Order and specificity of the *Plasmodium falciparum* hemoglobin degradation pathway. J. Clin. Invest. 93: 1602–1607

Goldberg, D. E., Slater, A. F. G. , Cerami, A., Henderson, G. B. (1990) Hemoglobin degradation in the malaria parasite *Plasmodium falciparum* : an ordered process in a unique organelle. Proc. Natl Acad. Sci. USA 87: 2931–2935

Hassan, H. F., Coombes, G. (1988) Purine and pyrimidine metabolism in parasitic protozoa. FEMS Microbiol. Rev. 743: 47–84

Hong, Y. L., Yang, Y. Z., Meshnick, S. R. (1994) The interaction of artemisinin with malarial hemozoin. Mol. Biochem. Parasitol. 63: 121–128

Hudson, A. T. (1993) Atovoquone – a novel broad-spectrum anti-infective drug. Parasitol. Today 9: 66–68

Hyde, J. E. (1989) Point mutations and pyrimethamine resistance in *Plasmodium falciparum*. Parasitol. Today 5: 252–255

Ivanetich, K. M., Santi, D. V. (1990) Thymidilate synthase-dihydrofolate reductase in protozoa. Exp. Parasitol. 70: 367–371

Krungkrai, S. R., Yuthavong, Y. (1987) The antimalarial action on *Plasmodium falciparum* of qinghaosu and artesunate in combination with agents which modulate oxidant stress. Trans. R. Soc. Trop. Med. Hyg. 81: 710–714

Krungkrai, J., Cerami, A., Henderson, G. B. (1990) Pyrimidine biosynthesis in parasitic protozoa: purification of a monofunctional dihydroorotatase from *Plasmodium berghei* and *Crithidia fasciculata*. Biochemistry 29: 6270–6275

Krungkrai, J., Krungkrai, S. R., Phakanont, K. (1992) Antimalarial activity of orotate analogs that inhibit dihydroorotase and dihydrorotate dehydrogenase. Biochem. Pharmacol. 17: 1295–1301

Kyle, D. E., Milhous, W. K., Rossan, R. N. (1993) Reversal of *Plasmodium falciparum* resistance to chloroquine in Panamanian Aotus monkey. Am. J. Trop. Med. Hyg. 48: 126–133

Meshnick, S. R. (1994) The mode of action of antimalarial endoperoxides. Trans. R. Soc. Trop. Med. Hyg. 88 (Suppl. 1): S31–S32

Meshnick, S. R., Yang, Y. Z., Lima, V., Kuypers, F., Kamchonwong-paisan, S., Yuthavong, Y. (1993) Iron-dependent free radical generation from the antimalarial agent artemisinin (qinghaosu). Antimicrob. Agents Chemother. 37: 1108–1114

Oduola, A. M., Omitowoju, G. O., Gerena, L., Kyle, D. E., Milhous, W. K., Sowunmi, A., Salako, L. A. (1993) Reversal of mefloquine resistance with penfluridol in isolates of *Plasmodium falciparum* from south-west Nigeria. Trans. R. Soc. Trop. Med. Hyg. 87: 81–83

Olliaro, P. L., Goldberg, D. E. (1995) The *Plasmodium* digestive vacuole: metabolic headquarters and choice drug target. Parasitol. Today 11: 294–297

Olliaro, P. L., Gottlieb, M. L., Wirth, D. F. (1996) *Plasmodium falciparum* proteinases: targeted drug development. Parasitol. Today 12: 413–414

Posner, G., Oh, C. H. (1992) A regiospecifically oxygen-18 labeled 1,2,4 trioxane: a simple chemical model to probe the mechanism(s) for the antimalarial activity of artemisinin (qinghaosu) J. Am. Chem. Soc. 114: 8328–8329

Posner, G. H., Oh, C. H., Webster, H. K., Ager Jr, A. L., Rossan, R. N. (1994) New, antimalarial, tricyclic 1,2,4-trioxanes: evaluations in mice and monkeys. Am. J. Trop. Med. Hyg. 50: 522–526

Posner, G. H., Wang, D., Gonzalez, L., Tao, X., Cumming, J. N., Klinedinst, D., Shapiro, T. A. (1996) Mechanism-based design of simple, symmetrical, easily prepared, potent antimalarial endoperoxides. Tetrahedron Lett. 37: 815–818

Peterson, D. S., Milhous, W. K., Wellems, T. E. (1990) Molecular basis of differential resistance to cycloguanil and pyrimethamine in *Plasmodium falciparum* malaria. Proc. Natl Acad. Sci. USA 87: 3018–3022

Rathod, P. K., Reyes, P. (1983) Orotidylate-metabolizing enzymes of the human malarial parasite, *Plasmodium falciparum*, differ from host cell enzymes. J. Biol. Chem. 258: 2852–2855

Ridley, R. G. (1997) Haemoglobin degradation and haem polymerization as antimalarial drug targets. J. Pharm. Pharmacol. 49(Suppl. 1):This issue

Rosenthal, P. J., Nelson, R. G. (1992) Isolation and characterization of a cysteine proteinase gene of *Plasmodium falciparum*. Mol. Biochem. Parasitol. 51: 143–152

Rosenthal, P. J., McKerrow, J. H., Aikawa, M., Nagasawa, H., Leech, J. H. D. (1988) A malarial cysteine proteinase is necessary for hemoglobin degradation by *Plasmodium falciparum*. J. Clin. Invest. 82: 1560–1566

Rosenthal, P. J., Wollish, W. S., Palmer, J. T., Rasnick, D. (1991) Antimalarial effects of peptide inhibitors of a *Plasmodium falciparum* cysteine proteinase. J. Clin. Invest. 88: 1467–1472

Rueenwongsa, P., Luanvararat, M., O'Sullivan, W. J. (1989) Serine hydroxymethyltransferase from pyrmethamine sensitive and -resistant strains of *Plasmodium chabaudi*. Mol. Biochem. Parasitol. 33: 265–272

Scheibel, L. W., Sherman, I. W. (1988) In: Wernsdorfer, W. H., McGregor, I. A. (eds) Malaria: Principles and Practice of Malariology. Vol 1, Churchill Livingstone, Edinburgh, pp 234–242

Seymour, K. K., Lyons, S. D., Phillips, L., Rieckmann, K. H., Christopherson, R. I. (1994) Cytotoxic effects of inhibitors of de novo pyrimidine biosynthesis upon *Plasmodium falciparum*. Biochemistry 33: 5268–5274

Slater, A. F. G., Cerami, A. (1992) Inhibition by chloroquine of a novel haem polymerase enzyme activity in malaria trophozoite. Nature 355: 167–169

Strath, M., Scott-Finnigan, T., Gardner, M., Williamson, D. H., Wilson, R. J. M. (1993) Antimalarial activity of rifampicin in vitro and in rodent malaria. Trans. R. Soc. Trop. Med. Hyg. 87: 211–216

Sullivan, D., Gluzman, I., Goldberg, D. (1996a) *Plasmodium* hemozoin formation mediated by histidine-rich proteins. Science 271: 219–222

Sullivan, D. J., Gluzman, I. Y., Russel, D. G., Goldberg, D. E. (1996b) On the molecular mechanism of chloroquine's antimalarial action. Proc. Natl Acad. Sci. USA (In press)

Vasanthakumar, G., Davis, R. L., Sullivan, M. A., Donahue, J. P. (1990) Cloning and expression of a hypoxanthine-guanine phosphoribosil transferase cDNA from *Plasmodium falciparum* in *E. coli*. Gene 91: 3587

Volkman, S. K., Wilson, C. M., Wirth, D. F. (1993) Stage-specific transcripts of *Plasmodium falciparum* pfmdr1 gene. Mol. Biochem. Parasitol. 57: 203–212

Wilson, R. J. M., Gardner, M. J., Feagin, J. E., Williamson, D..H. (1991) Have malaria parasites three genomes? Parasitol. Today 7: 134–136

Wilson, C. M., Volkman, S. K., Thaithong, S., Martin, R. K., Kyle, D. S., Milhous, W. K., Wirth, D. F. (1993) Amplification of pfmdr1 associated with mefloquine and halofantrine resistance in *Plasmodium falciparum* in Thailand. Mol. Biochem. Parasitol. 57: 151–160

Yang, Y. Z., Little, B., Meshnick, S. R. (1993) Alkylation of proteins by artemisinin. Effects of heme, pH, and drug structure. Biochem. Pharmacol. 48: 569–573

Zhao, Y., Kappes, B., Franklin, M. (1993) Gene structure and expression of an unusual protein kinase from *Plasmodium falciparum* homologous at tiscarboxyl terminus with the EF hand calcium-binding proteins. J. Biol. Chem. 268: 4347–4354

J. Pharm. Pharmacol. 1997, 49 (Suppl. 2): 35–41

Mediators and Mechanisms Associated with Paroxysm in *Plasmodium vivax* Malaria

R. CARTER, S. K. WIJESEKERA*, N. D. KARUNAWEERA* AND K. N. MENDIS*

*Division of Biological Sciences, ICAPB, University of Edinburgh, Edinburgh EH9 3JT, UK, and *University of Colombo, Faculty of Medicine, Malaria Research Unit, Colombo 8, Sri Lanka*

The Clinical Manifestations and Biological Basis of Paroxysm and its Relationship to Other Malaria Pathology

The paroxysm of human malaria is most clearly expressed in infections with that species of parasite whose effects were recognized in early times as "benign tertian" fevers and which, since the end of the last century, has been known as *Plasmodium vivax*. Infections with *P. vivax* were termed benign, or as would be said today, uncomplicated, in distinction from the severe morbidity and occasional mortality associated with infections due to the other highly prevalent species of human malaria, *Plasmodium falciparum*. The severe pathologies of *P. falciparum* infection involve organ dysfunction (e.g. cerebral malaria, renal failure, severe anaemia) and often irreversible tissue damage. The pathology of *P. vivax* infections, on the other hand, is almost invariably transient and with no detectable tissue damaging consequences. The symptoms of *P. vivax* infection are malaise, anorexia and tendency to prostration with periodic episodes of acute fever which may be accompanied by headache, nausea and vomiting and moderate to severe muscle, joint and back pain.

Neither the physiological basis of the severe and complicated pathologies found among *P. falciparum* infections, nor that of the benign pathology of paroxysm in *P. vivax* infections are understood. There are, however, biological differences between the parasites which certainly account, at least in part, for their different pathological manifestations. Thus in *P. falciparum* infection there is invariable sequestration of the maturing asexual blood-stage parasites by ligand-mediated attachment to the endothelial lining of the post-capillary microvasculature. This results in virtually continuous aggravation of the endothelial tissues in every organ affected and presumably contributes, in the minority of cases, to induction of the mediators of severe pathology.

By contrast, *P. vivax* blood-stage parasites do not sequester to any detectable degree at any stage in their development. Being intracellular parasites of red blood cells (RBC) their presence in the body is registered and responded to, particularly following the period of schizont rupture, an event which occurs synchronously at almost exactly 48-h intervals (or, as not infrequently occurs, at 24-h intervals when two distinct broods of the parasites are present in the blood). The first 2–3 rounds of schizont rupture, following release of the parasites in the blood from the sporozoite-induced (mosquito-inoculated) liver stage of the infection, are largely asymptomatic (the prodromal period). Thereafter, the full-blown clinical symp-

toms of a paroxysm are suddenly manifest following the next schizont rupture event, usually when parasite densities are still less than one parasitized RBC per 100 000 uninfected RBCs.

The first symptoms of a *P. vivax* paroxysm, which are felt within 1–2 h after the beginning of schizont rupture, are a sudden feeling of chill; within a few minutes the victim takes to bed and seeks to cover him or herself with a sheet or blanket, adopting a hunched or foetal position. Within 5–10 min the sufferer is shaking with considerable violence and, although experiencing a sensation of great cold, is in fact undergoing a steep rise in body temperature. What has happened is that the body's thermostat has been reset to several degrees above normal accounting for both the sensation of cold and for the rising temperature as the body adjusts to reach the reset level. About 1 h after the first feeling of chill, the victim looses the cold sensation and one of internal warmth returns soon proceeding to one of high fever, the bed clothes being cast aside in an attempt to lose heat. Headache, muscle, joint and back pains may now become prominent and even severe; nausea and vomiting may occur. Within 3–4 h after onset, the temperature, which peaks typically at 39–40°C, begins to fall; this is usually accompanied by profuse sweating which can leave the bedclothes literally drenched with perspiration. As other symptoms slowly remit, the exhausted sufferer may fall into peaceful sleep perhaps 4–6 h after the onset. Within 8–10 h the temperature has returned to normal.

This account would be typical of a paroxysm in a non-immune sufferer. The exact picture can vary, especially in the associated symptoms. However, the chill, rigor (shaking) and soaring temperature are almost invariably experienced. The mediators and mechanisms of the paroxysm of *P. vivax* malaria are certainly different from those of the severe pathologies associated with *P. falciparum* malaria. Nevertheless, experimental investigations and speculation have identified certain substances of host or parasite origin as being generally implicated in malarial disease. Prominent among these are the cytokine tumour necrosis factor alpha (TNFα) (Clark et al 1992) and the products of the parasites released during schizont rupture (Kwiatkowski 1995).

TNFα has long been the subject of investigations which have sought to define it in a causative role in the severe and complicated pathologies of *P. falciparum* malaria, notably in cerebral malaria. While several studies have shown an association between circulating TNFα levels and severity of disease in *P. falciparum* malaria (Grau et al 1989; Kern et al 1989; Kwiatkowski et al 1990), there are no experiments which demonstrate a direct causal relationship between the activity of this cytokine and severe pathology in malaria. An experimental clinical intervention in severe malaria cases with an anti-TNFα monoclonal antibody did not protect against fatal outcome

Correspondence: R Carter, Division of Biological Sciences, ICAPB, The University of Edinburgh, West Mains Road, Edinburgh EH9 3JN, UK.

(Kwiatkowski et al 1993) but did, on the other hand, achieve significant reduction in fever. Consistent with a role for TNFα as a key pyrogen in malarial infection is the finding that circulating levels of the cytokine in cases of *P. vivax* malaria rose sharply at the onset of a paroxysm and declined in close parallel with the fall in temperature after the paroxysm (Karunaweera et al 1992b) (Fig. 1). Moreover, the circulating levels of TNFα during paroxysms in *P. vivax* infections often exceeded those seen in the severest cases of *P. falciparum* malaria. Thus the circumstantial evidence is consistent with the role of TNFα as an endogenous pyrogen of malarial fevers but mitigates against TNFα as a sole and sufficient mediator of severe pathology of *P. falciparum* malaria.

The other class of mediators of malaria pathology which has received much attention is represented by the parasite products released following schizont rupture. The concept of a malaria toxin must have arisen in the minds of the early malariologists and it acquired a specific biological context when it was discovered that the periodic fevers of malaria are co-ordinated with the synchronous rupture of the blood stage schizonts of the parasites. This relationship was investigated experimentally by a working party of the United States Public Health Service at Vera Cruz in Mexico in 1904 (Rosenau et al 1905). These workers demonstrated that the full blown symptoms of a *P. vivax* paroxysm could be passively transferred to a healthy individual by intravenous injection of serum taken at the height of a paroxysm from a *P. vivax* sufferer; serum taken at times other than during the paroxysm had no effect on a recipient. In

their report of these experiments the investigators were cautious not to claim discovery of the malaria toxin itself. This was wise, as we now realize that other mediators, such as TNFα itself, could have been, and probably were, directly responsible for the effect. Nevertheless, the experiments proved that potent pyrogens were transiently present shortly after the rupture of the blood-stage schizonts and, while admiring the caution of these American workers, it would be hard not to conclude from their experiments that the products of the schizont rupture were either the pyrogens themselves, the inducers of the pyrogens or both the inducers and, in some synergistic way, the co-mediators with those they had induced, of the febrile and other events of the paroxysm.

Recent investigations with the products of schizonts of malaria parasites prepared in-vitro, have shown that these products are, indeed, potent stimuli of TNFα production by human peripheral blood monocytes in culture (Bate et al 1992; Allan et al 1993). There is now significant literature which has explored the nature of the parasite products which are involved in such TNFα induction (Playfair et al 1990; Mendis & Carter 1995; Kwiatkowski 1995). There is general agreement that these products are glycolipid in nature, do not involve protein in their activity and, by antigenic criteria and biological activity, cannot be readily distinguished between different species of malaria parasite, including the two human species *P. falciparum* and *P. vivax*.

While no-one, today, can claim comprehensive insight into the mechanisms of malaria pathogenesis, the following general scenarios for the involvement of soluble mediators are commonly at the centre of contemporary investigation and discussion.

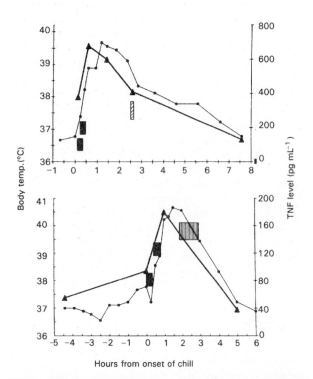

FIG. 1. Body temperature (measured orally) (●), plasma TNF level (▲) and the period and duration of the chill (hatched box), rigor (black box) and sweating (grey box) during the course of a single paroxysm in two of the nine *P. vivax* patients studied. The parallel between changes in body temperature and plasma TNF levels was as close as is shown here in eight of the nine patients studied. Reproduced by permission of the Proceedings of the National Academy of Sciences, USA (Karunaweera et al 1992b).

Severe pathology

TNFα, induced by parasite products, perhaps locally at the sites of deep vascular sequestration, acts secondarily on local tissues, e.g. venous endothelium, to up-regulate expression of ligands involved in binding of parasitized RBCs and parasite sequestration, and to induce secondary mediators such as nitric oxide or oxygen free radicals, or both, which inflict direct organ-malfunction and tissue damage.

Paroxysm (non-severe pathology)

Parasite products released into the blood circulation at the time of schizont rupture induce circulating monocytes to produce TNFα and possibly other pyrogenic cytokines, IL-1 and IL-6, which act on the thermoregulatory centre in the hypothalamus to reset the body thermostat and induce the fever of paroxysm.

As already stated there is apparent overlap between the general hypotheses for malarial paroxysm and for severe pathology in malaria in that both invoke the induction of TNFα by the action of parasite products on (it is generally assumed) blood monocytes. If this is, indeed, a true representation of the two very different types of pathological condition, it will require detailed investigation of the other mechanisms involved to achieve an understanding of why the clinical manifestations are so different. In seeking to understand the basis of malaria pathogenesis we have devoted the investigations presented here to exploring the mechanisms of the paroxysm of *P. vivax* malaria.

The Biological Significance of the Paroxysm of *P. vivax* Malaria

In the early stages of a malarial, or indeed any, blood infection in a previously unexposed host, it has been generally assumed that there can have been no time for an effective pathogen antigen-specific protective immune response to mature. The host is, therefore, presumed to be dependent for the prevention of uncontrolled parasitic infestation, upon its ability to mount innate, parasite density-controlling responses. As has been pointed out (Kwiatkowski 1995), such a response, in a human host, to the early stages of malarial infection can be reasonably argued to be represented by the paroxysm of malaria, of which the role of high body temperature in killing malaria parasites has been emphasized. In the case of malaria it appears that the mature forms of the parasite are those most sensitive to high temperature as has been demonstrated in-vitro (Kwiatkowski 1989). As a consequence, the fever of paroxysm presumably has the effect not only of culling the parasites but of doing so by eliminating all but the youngest parasites newly invaded into red blood cells. Since it is the most mature forms of the parasites, the rupturing schizonts, which initiate the paroxysm, the net effect is to tightly synchronize the blood infection by leaving only the youngest parasites alive shortly after schizont rupture. While the temperature sensitivity of mature asexual blood-stage malaria parasites, and indeed of mature malaria gametocytes, can be readily demonstrated in-vitro, the parasite-killing effects of paroxysm in-vivo have been taken on faith. Some observations made in our laboratory in Sri Lanka on the infectivity of naturally acquired primary infections of *P. vivax* to mosquitoes, however, provide direct evidence that such an effect may occur during a malarial paroxysm. Thus, mosquitoes became infected when fed on the arms of *P. vivax*-infected volunteers when they were without symptoms but those fed on the same patients during a paroxysm almost invariably failed to acquire infection (unpublished data).

This observation suggested that blood-stage parasites were indeed being killed or inactivated during malarial paroxysm and raised the question as to whether the infectious stages, the gametocytes, were being inactivated only by the fever itself or whether other factors were involved. To test this question we collected plasmas from *P. vivax* patients during the peak of their paroxysms. We then collected *P. vivax*-infected blood from volunteers who were without symptoms, and whose gametocytes were in an infectious state. The infectious gametocytes were cultured in-vitro for 3 h with medium containing paroxysmal plasma and subsequently resuspended in normal serum and fed to mosquitoes through a membrane. Almost invariably it was found that the infectivity of the gametocytes pre-incubated in the paroxysm plasmas was reduced by 70 to 80% compared to that of equivalent samples of the same gametocyte-infected blood pre-incubated in normal plasmas from healthy control donors (Karunaweera et al 1992a). Plasmas drawn a few hours before the onset of a paroxysm and plasmas drawn following its resolution had only a slight suppressive effect on the infectivity of the gametocytes to mosquitoes (Karunaweera et al 1992a; Wijesekera et al 1996).

These results showed that, independent of any effects due to temperature, there are active substances present in plasma during a paroxysm that mediate the suppression of gametocyte infectivity to mosquitoes. Moreover, the parasite-inactivating mediators are rapidly induced around the time of onset of the paroxysm, and, with similar rapidity, cease to be effective after the paroxysm has passed.

It was evident that the experimental system which we had devised to test the effects of plasma on the infectivity of gametocyte-infected blood to mosquitoes, was, in fact, a precise assay for the presence of some, as yet undefined, mediators whose activity coincided exactly with the period of a paroxysm of *P. vivax* malaria. The investigations summarised in this article are from studies, using this assay, on mediators and mechanisms within the circulating blood cells and plasma during the clinical event of paroxysm.

Investigations on the Paroxysm of *P. vivax* Malaria

Gametocyte inactivation by P. vivax *paroxysm plasma depends upon the presence of blood monocytes and appears to be mediated, at least in part, by nitric oxide*

In order to test whether the activities of soluble mediators, whose presence we deduced in the paroxysm plasmas, were dependent upon the presence of nucleated blood cells, we conducted the following experiments. Before incubating *P. vivax* gametocyte-infected blood cells with paroxysm plasma, we depleted the cells either of T cells (with antibodies to the pan T-cell surface antigen CD2, conjugated to magnetic beads—Dynabeads from Dynal) or of monocytes (with Dynabead-conjugated antibodies to the CD14 antigen – which has, in fact, been identified as the endotoxin receptor of these cells). Depletion of T cells was without effect on the activity of the paroxysm plasma; depletion of the monocytes, on the other hand, removed the effect almost completely. Thus the active factors in the paroxysm plasmas that mediated suppression of gametocyte infectivity, were totally dependent for their effect upon the presence of peripheral blood monocytes (unpublished data).

Data from other studies have indicated that the inactivation of malaria gametocytes by activated white blood cells is mediated by nitric oxide (NO) (Naotunne et al 1993).

The activity of P. vivax *paroxysm plasma is totally dependent upon the presence of the cytokine TNFα and upon the presence of products which can be neutralized by antibodies against* P. vivax *antigens*

As discussed above, there are two types of mediator which might immediately be suspected to have a role in a monocyte-mediated activity co-incident with the paroxysm of malaria. They are the products of the parasites themselves acting as endotoxin, and the cytokine TNFα, the prime candidate for the endogenous pyrogen in the paroxysm of malaria. These possibilities were tested by pre-incubating paroxysm plasma with antibodies raised in rabbits against extracts of *P. vivax* schizonts and with a neutralizing monoclonal antibody against human TNFα. Both treatments completely removed the activity of the paroxysm plasmas, indicating that both TNFα and parasite products were essential to induce monocytes to inactivate *P. vivax* gametocytes (Karunaweera et al 1992a; Wijesekera et al 1996).

These results are entirely compatible with the favoured view of malaria paroxysm which envisages that parasite products released at schizogony act as an endotoxin to induce circulating blood monocytes to produce TNFα and that this cytokine

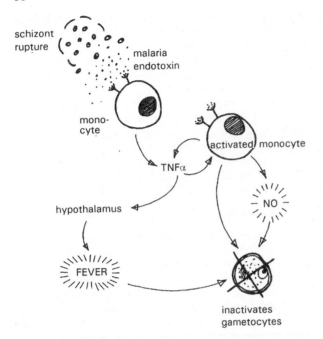

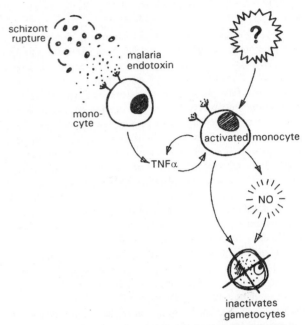

FIG. 2.   Scheme representing cellular events and mediators during a *Plasmodium vivax* paroxysm.

FIG. 3.   Scheme representing cellular events and mediators during a *Plasmodium vivax* paroxysm showing that Fig. 2 does not fully account for the parasite-killing activity of the blood monocytes during a paroxysm.

is the endogenous pyrogen which mediates the induction of the clinical events of the paroxysm (Fig. 2). The next set of experiments, however, showed that this is not a sufficient description of the mediators and mechanisms which must be involved, at least as regards the gametocyte inactivating effects of paroxysm plasma.

Parasite products and TNFα are not sufficient to induce human blood monocytes to carry out gametocyte inactivation
If TNFα and parasite products were all that were necessary to induce blood monocytes to mediate the inactivation of *P. vivax* gametocytes, then it should be possible to induce such inactivation by addition of these to normal human plasma. Such addition, however, was totally without effect on the infectivity of *P. vivax* gametocyte-infected blood (Wijesekera et al 1996). On the other hand, their addition to plasma drawn shortly after a paroxysm (which of itself has little or no effect on the infectivity of gametocyte-infected blood) caused the post paroxysm plasma to bring about potent inactivation of the gametocytes (Wijesekera et al 1996). Addition of the parasite extracts and TNFα to plasmas drawn just before a paroxysm had a moderate but much lower effect (unpublished data).

These results proved that there are additional factors, absent in normal human plasma, which begin to appear in plasma from just before a paroxysm and which are highly active in plasma immediately following a paroxysm. The parasite products and TNFα are absolutely dependent upon these factors to be able to induce blood monocytes to mediate gametocyte inactivation (Fig. 3).

Activation of monocytes to suppress infectivity of gametocytes to mosquitoes during a paroxysm is absolutely dependent upon the presence of IL-2 and GM-CSF
To search for the unidentified mediator(s) upon which the monocytes were dependent to suppress gametocyte infectivity

during a *P. vivax* paroxysm, we tested the effects of neutralizing antibodies against most of the remaining human cytokines for which such reagents were available. Of these, including antibodies to IL-1α and β, IL-6 and IFNγ, only antibodies against IL-2 and GM-CSF (granulocyte–macrophage-colony stimulating factor), mediated reversal of the effects of paroxysm plasma (unpublished data). IL-2 is the product, virtually exclusively, of activated T cells and of no other cell type (except NK cells) and GM-CSF is a maturation-stimulatory cytokine which acts on macrophages/monocytes, neutrophils and eosinophils and which is the product of T cells, B cells and monocytes.

To test the involvement of IL-2, we reconstituted normal human plasma with parasite extract and TNFα (a combination which we had previously shown does not induce monocytes to inactivate gametocytes) and added, in addition, IL-2. This combination now induced monocyte-dependent inactivation of *P. vivax* gametocytes as effectively as did paroxysm plasma itself (unpublished data). Confirmation that this almost uniquely T-cell-derived mediator, IL-2, is essential to recreate the effects of paroxysm plasma, leads us to the hypothesis that the parasite-killing aspect of monocyte activation during a malaria paroxysm is under the direct control of activated T cells (Fig. 4).

The cellular origin of the GM-CSF in the paroxysm plasma is uncertain at this stage; it could be either a monocyte or a T-cell product, or both. Its likely function in the parasite killing events would be to activate monocytes and granulocytes around the location of the parasitized cells.

The parasite products in paroxysm plasma which induce white blood cells to inactivate gametocytes are antigenically distinct and parasite species-specific
Immune sera raised in rabbits against freeze-thawed extracts of the blood-stage schizonts of either *P. vivax* or *P. falciparum*

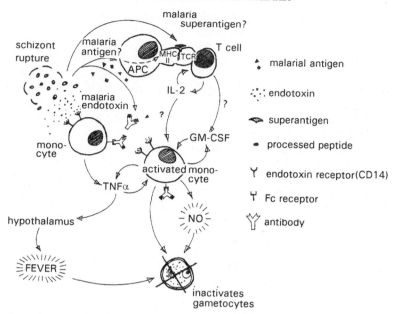

FIG. 4. Scheme representing the putative role of antigen-activated T cells and of parasite antigens in the activation of monocytes during a paroxysm of *Plasmodium vivax* malaria.

have been tested for their ability to reverse the ability of *P. vivax* paroxysm plasma to inactivate gametocytes of this parasite. Paroxysm plasma to which antisera against *P. vivax* extracts were added no longer suppressed infectivity of gametocyte-infected blood to mosquitoes. Antisera against extracts of blood schizonts of *P. falciparum*, on the other hand, were completely without effect (Wijesekera et al 1996). These findings indicate that the parasite products in paroxysm plasma which are active in stimulating the anti-parasitic activity of the white blood cells are species-specific antigens of their respective parasites.

This result stands in striking contrast to the evidence that the parasite products which induce TNF from monocytes in-vitro are antigenically indistinguishable between the two species of parasite (Bate et al 1992).

Discussion

Our investigations have enabled us to define and follow the effects of soluble mediators elaborated during the paroxysm of *P. vivax* malaria. We have used an assay which monitors the ability of peripheral blood monocytes to suppress the infectivity of gametocytes of the parasites to mosquitoes; this is, in effect, an assay of monocyte-mediated parasite killing during paroxysm.

We have shown that the active mediators of monocyte-dependent gametocyte inactivation present in paroxysm plasma include products of the parasites themselves, presumably released during schizont rupture preceding the paroxysm. Another essential mediator in activation of the monocytes is the cytokine TNFα. This cytokine is known to reach high levels during a paroxysm and is probably also the key endogenous pyrogen responsible for the induction of the clinical events of a paroxysm. It is also clear from our results, that the anti-parasitic activity of monocytes during a paroxysm, is absolutely dependent upon the presence of the activated T-cell product IL-2. Moreover, this factor becomes active no

sooner than the onset of a clinical paroxysm, a fact which can be reasonably accounted for only if the T cells are activated to secrete IL-2 by parasite products released at the time of the schizont rupture.

If this conclusion is correct we can no longer regard all the events which take place during a paroxysm as simply the reflex, or innate, response of blood monocytes to the abrupt release of a parasite-derived endotoxin. At least certain aspects of these events, namely those involved in cell-mediated killing of the parasites, are now seen to fall under the control of antigen-activated T cells. There are two general possibilities for the nature of the putative antigen–T-cell relationship involved.

One possible way of explaining the activation of the T cells is to invoke the existence of malaria superantigen. Superantigens have been described from certain micro-organisms, notably *Staphlococcus aureus* B enterotoxin; their distinctive immunologic feature is that they cross-link between a major histocompatibility complex (MHC) II molecule and a T cell receptor, not by binding in the groove of the MHC molecule as do the processed peptides of conventional protein antigens, but by binding across the outer faces of the two molecules. Superantigens are able to interact with about 10–20% of a T-cell population. If this were the basis of T-cell activation during paroxysm there would be no necessity for T-cell priming by prior exposure to antigen. A paroxysm would presumably be initiated once the blood parasites passed some critical lower threshold for recognition. As far as we are aware, however, there is no evidence that malaria parasites possess material having superantigen type properties (Jones et al 1990).

The alternative is that the T cells are recognizing and responding to parasite products processed by antigen-presenting cells through conventional pathways and presented in association with an MHC class II molecule for recognition by an antigen-specific, MHC-restricted T-cell receptor. Such a scenario would require the priming and expansion of antigen-specific T-cell clones by previous exposure to the malarial antigens. The lag that would be involved in generating such expanded antigen-specific clones could account for the pro-dromal period during which two to three rounds of parasite replication occur in the blood without inducing clinical symptoms in the naive individual. It is also possible that these antigens are acting on T-cell clones that have been previously primed and expanded by cross-reacting antigens of non-malarial origin (Currier et al 1995).

We have also found that the monocyte-mediated inactiva-tion of gametocytes induced by *P. vivax* paroxysm plasma, can be reversed by immune sera raised against schizonts of *P. vivax* but not by immune sera raised against schizonts of *P. falciparum*. This finding, however, does not seem to relate to the antigens which activate T cells to produce IL-2 during a paroxysm. We can state this because IL-2 is already active in paroxysm plasma, but the parasite-killing effect of the plasma is still totally dependent upon the presence of the species-specific antigens. It is possible that these antigens are in fact endotoxins, although this rather complicates the evidence from other findings that the endotoxin of malaria is not species-specific (Bate et al 1992). Another possibility could be that the species-specific antigens activate monocytes in the form of complexes with cytophilic antibodies (Fig. 4). Antimalarial antibodies can, in fact, be detected in the serum of malaria-infected persons at the time their plasma shows parasite killing effects during a paroxysm (unpublished observations).

It is a notable consequence of these hypotheses that aspects of what has usually been represented to be an innate, non-cognitive, response to early parasitization—namely the par-oxysm of malaria—may, be controlled by antigen-specific cognate immune processes.

If this situation is true, it is also probable that the parasite products, or antigens, to which the paroxysm-controlling T cells respond, and also the hypothetical monocyte-activating, immune-complexed, species-specific antigens in paroxysm plasma, are of different chemical composition to the endo-toxin-like product responsible for TNFα induction by periph-eral blood cells in-vitro (Dick et al 1996). As already mentioned, results from such in-vitro investigations upon endotoxin-like products of blood-stage malaria schizonts sug-gest that these are glycolipid in nature, do not involve protein and are antigenically similar between different species of malaria parasites. A product which activates T cells via con-ventional MHC antigen presentation is, virtually by definition, a protein. If the antigens which prime and activate the T cells which control *P. vivax* paroxysms are protein, then it is almost certain that the relevant molecules are also antigenically dis-tinct between different species of malaria parasite. Likewise, the active parasite products whose presence we have detected in the paroxysm plasma are antigenically distinct and species-specific; these too may well be proteins. Our experiments provide no direct evidence that the monocyte-mediated, T cell–IL-2-controlled events of parasite-killing (gametocyte inacti-vation) that take place during a *P. vivax* paroxysm are causally related to the induction of the clinical symptoms of the par-oxysm. It would, indeed, be quite consistent with our present data to postulate that a purely endotoxin-dependent induction of TNFα was responsible for the clinical symptoms of parox-ysm. The parasite-killing events, whose mediators and com-ponents we have investigated, could thus represent an almost

entirely separate, but concurrent, sequence of events having only the common cause of schizont rupture and the release of active parasite products to connect it with the clinical experi-ence of the paroxysm. There could, on the other hand, be close causal linkage between the initiators and mediators of the parasite-killing and clinical events of paroxysm. Experience with the use of IL-2 therapy in cancer patients has shown that this cytokine, central to the events that we have described in association with paroxysm, induces a malaria-like paroxysm with chill and high fever about 2 hours following its admin-istration. Investigation of the phenomenon showed that the IL-2 was not itself a pyrogen but that it rapidly induced pyrogenic activity which could be entirely accounted for by the presence of TNFα (Mier et al 1988). These findings bear obvious rele-vance to the possible interpretations of our own.

The hypotheses which we have presented from our data, that events associated with the paroxysm of *P. vivax* malaria are under the control of (presumably antigen-specific) T cells, and that species-specific antigens are involved in the immediate activation of paroxysm-associated, parasite-killing events, may be relevant to the regulation of other types of pathogenesis in malaria and, indeed, to anti-blood-stage immunity to malaria in general. It is striking that the immuno-physiological responses of the host during a paroxysm of *P. vivax* malaria are essen-tially anti-parasitic and, however acutely distressing to the infected host, result in little or no permanent tissue damage. It is interesting to contrast this situation with the destructive pathologies that can arise during *P. falciparum* infections and to speculate upon the mediators and their control, or lack of it, which may be involved.

Acknowledgements

These studies by our groups at the University of Colombo and at the University of Edinburgh have been supported at various times by the Rockefeller Foundation, the World Health Organization TDR Programme and the EC or EU STD Pro-gramme and the Medical Research Council of the UK. Our thanks also to Eleanor Riley for helpful comments on this manuscript.

References

Allan, R. J., Rowe, A., Kwiatkowski, D. (1993) *Plasmodium falci-parum* varies in its ability to induce tumour necrosis factor. Infect. Immun. 61: 4772–4776

Bate, C. A. W., Taverne, J., Karunaweera, N. D., Mendis, K. N., Kwiatkowski, D., Playfair, J. H. L. (1992) Serological relationship of tumour necrosis factor-inducing exoantigens of *Plasmodium falciparum* and *Plasmodium vivax*. Infect. Immun. 60: 1241–1243

Clark, I. A., Rockett, K. A., Cowden, W. B. (1992) TNF in malaria. In: Beutler, B. (ed.) Tumour Necrosis Factor: The Molecules and Their Emerging Role in Medicine. Raven Press, New York, p. 303

Currier, J., Beck, H. P., Currie, B., Good, M. F. (1995) Antigens released at schizont burst stimulate *Plasmodium falciparum* – specific CD4(+) T-cells from non-exposed donors – potential for cross-reactive memory T-cells to cause disease. Int. Immunol. 7: 821–833

Dick, S., Waterfall, M., Currie, J., Maddy, A., Riley, E. (1996) Naive human αβT cells respond to membrane-associated components of malaria-infected erythrocytes by proliferation and production of interferon-γ. Immunol. 88: 412–420

Grau, G. E., Taylor, T. E., Molineux, M. E., Wirima, J. T., Vasselli, P., Hommel, M., Lambert, P. H. (1989) Tumour necrosis factor and disease severity in children with falciparum malaria. N. Engl. J. Med. 320: 1586–1591

Jones, K. R., Hickling, J. K., Targett, G. A. T., Playfair, J. H. L. (1990) Polyclonal in vitro proliferative responses from non-immune donors to *Plasmodium falciparum* malaria antigens require UCHL1 + (memory) T cells. Eur. J. Immunol. 20: 307–310

Karunaweera, N. D., Carter, R., Grau, G. E., Kwiatkowski, D., Del Giudice, G., Mendis, K. N. (1992a) Tumour necrosis factor-dependent parasite-killing effects during paroxysms in non-immune *Plasmodium vivax* malaria patients. Clin. Exp. Immunol. 88: 499–505

Karunaweera, N. D., Grau,G. E., Gamage, P., Carter, R., Mendis, K. N. (1992b) Dynamics of fever and serum TNF levels are closely associated during clinical paroxysms in *Plasmodium vivax* malaria. Proc. Natl Acad. Sci. USA 89: 3200–3203

Kern, P., Hemmer, C. J., Vandamme, J., Gruss, H. J., Dietrich, M. (1989) Elevated tumour necrosis factor-alpha and interleukin-6 serum levels as markers for complicated *Plasmodium falciparum* malaria. Am. J. Med. 87: 139–143

Kwiatkowski, D. (1989) Febrile temperatures can synchronize the growth of *Plasmodium falciparum* in vitro. J. Exp. Med. 169: 357–361

Kwiatkowski, D. (1995) Malaria toxins and the regulation of parasite density. Parasitol. Today 11: 206–212

Kwiatkowski, D., Cannon, J. G., Manogue, K. R., Cerami, A., Dinarello, C. A., Greenwood, B. M. (1989) Tumour necrosis factor production in falciparum-malaria and its association with schizont rupture. Clin. Exp. Immunol. 77: 361–366

Kwiatkowski, D., Hill, A. V. S., Sambou, I., Twumasi, P., Castracane, J., Manogue, K. R., Cerami, A., Brewster, D. R., Greenwood, B. M. (1990) TNF concentrations in fatal cerebral, nonfatal cerebral, and uncomplicated *Plasmodium-falciparum* malaria. Lancet 336: 1201–1204

Kwiatkowski, D., Molineux, M. E., Stephens, S., Curtis, N., Klein, N., Pointaire, P., Smit, M., Allan, R., Brewster, D. R., Grau, G. E., Greenwood, B. M. (1993) Anti-TNF therapy inhibits fever in cerebral malaria. Quart. J. Med. 86: 91–98

Mendis, K. N., Carter, R. (1995) Clinical Disease and Pathogenesis in Malaria. Parasitol. Today 11: 1–16

Mier, J. W., Vachino, G., Van Der Meer, J. W. M., Numerof, R. P, Adams, A., Cannon, J. G., Bernheim, H. A., Atkins, M. B., Parkinson, D. R., Dinarello, C. A. (1988) Induction of circulating tumour necrosis factor (TNFα) as the mechanism for the febrile response to Interleukin-2 (IL-2) in cancer patients. J. Clin. Immunol. 8: 426–436

Naotunne, T. de S., Karunaweera, N. D., Mendis, K. N., Carter, R. (1993) Cytokine-mediated inactivation of malarial gametocytes is dependent on the presence of white blood cells and involves reactive nitrogen intermediates. Immunol. 78: 555–562

Playfair, J. H. L., Taverne, J., Bate, C. A. W., DeSouza, J. B. (1990) The malaria vaccine – antiparasitic or antidisease. Immunol. Today 11: 25–27

Rosenau, M. J., Parker, H. B., Francis,E., Beyer, G. E. (1905) Report of Working Party No. 2, Yellow Fever Institute. Experimental studies in Yellow Fever and Malaria at Vera Cruz, Mexico, Yellow Fever Institute, Bulletin No. 14, Washington Government Printing Office, pp 49–101

Wijesekera, S. K., Carter, R. Rathnayaka, L., Mendis, K. N. (1996) A malaria parasite toxin associated with *Plasmodium vivax* paroxysms. Clin. Exp. Immunol. 104: 221–227

J. Pharm. Pharmacol. 1997, 49 (Suppl. 2): 43-48

Haemoglobin Degradation and Haem Polymerization as Antimalarial Drug Targets

ROBERT G. RIDLEY

F. Hoffmann-La Roche, Pharmaceuticals Division, Pharma Research, CH-4070 Basel, Switzerland

To assist in the discovery of new classes of antimalarial compounds, and to thus ensure the long-term future of antimalarial drug development, it is essential to better characterize parasite cell biology at the molecular level. The best antimicrobial drug targets involve cellular processes that are both unique and essential for the organism. The obligate requirement of malarial parasites to reside inside the host's erythrocytes, and their dependence, during this stage of their life cycle, on the ingestion and degradation of haemoglobin represents such a critical process (Olliaro & Goldberg 1995). Proteases involved in haemoglobin degradation, and the sequestration of the toxic haem generated as a result, are the subject of the chemotherapeutic approaches outlined in this article.

The Biology of Haemoglobin Degradation

The degradation of haemoglobin takes place in an acidic lysosomal organelle called the digestive vacuole (Olliaro & Goldberg 1995). Estimates of the amount of haemoglobin degraded during the parasite's occupancy of the host erythrocyte has varied from 25 to 80% (Ball et al 1948; Groman 1951; Roth et al 1986). The reasons for this high level of metabolic activity are probably two-fold. Firstly, the amino acids released from haemoglobin are a potential source of nutrients. This is supported by evidence that parasite growth in culture requires supplementation with amino acids (methionine, cysteine, isoleucine, glutamine and glutamate) that are absent or of low abundance in haemoglobin (Divo et al 1985; Francis et al 1994). Secondly, the parasite requires space to grow and develop in the erythrocyte and may need to degrade haemoglobin to achieve this. This is supported by evidence that not all the products of haemoglobin degradation are required by the parasite (Vander Jagt et al 1992). Reconstitution of erythrocytes containing as little as 6% of the original haemoglobin can support parasite growth (Rangachari et al 1987) and a large proportion of the amino acids generated by haemoglobin degradation are secreted from the parasite (Zarchin et al 1986).

Several types of protease are involved in haemoglobin degradation. Using specific inhibitors to study haemoglobin degradation in-vitro, aspartic protease, cysteine protease, serine protease and metalloprotease activities have all been detected in digestive vacuole extracts (Goldberg et al 1990). However, only two aspartic proteinases (plasmepsins I and II) and one cysteine proteinase (falcipain) have been characterized at the molecular level. These are discussed in detail later.

Correspondence: R. G. Ridley, Pharmaceuticals Division, Pharma Research Pre-clinical Infectious Diseases (PRPI), F. Hoffmann-La Roche, CH-4070 Basel, Switzerland. E-Mail: robert_g.ridley@roche.com

Degradation of haemoglobin releases ferrous (iron II) haem. This powerful reducing agent is a generator of free radicals, which are thought to be inactivated in the food vacuole by peroxidases and superoxide dismutases (Olliaro & Goldberg 1995). In the presence of peroxide antimalarial drugs, such as artemisinin, free radical derivatives and other reactive derivatives of the drugs are generated (Haynes & Vonwiller 1996; Posner 1997). These cannot be inactivated and are lethal for the malarial parasite, probably due to alkylation of proteins, lipids and other cellular components (Meshnick et al 1996).

The ferric (iron III) haematin resulting from the oxidation of ferrous (iron II) haem remains toxic for the parasite, as it is membrane interactive and potentially lytic (Fitch et al 1982, 1983). In many organisms, haem moieties are degraded by a haem oxygenase system (Schacter 1988), but such a process operating in the food vacuole would probably result in greater oxidative stress for the parasite. Instead, the monomeric iron III haematin is detoxified by polymerization into a form of polymeric β-haematin called haemozoin, or malaria pigment (Slater et al 1991; Bohle et al 1994). It is believed that inhibition of haem polymerization is lethal for the parasite.

A schematic representation of the process of haemoglobin degradation operating in the digestive vacuole is shown in Fig. 1. The potential of haem polymerization, and the proteinases involved in haemoglobin degradation, as targets for chemotherapy are explored in more detail in the following sections.

Inhibition of Haem Polymerization

Haem polymerization was originally thought to be an enzyme-mediated process (Slater & Cerami 1992). However, it was later demonstrated that the original activity observed was protein independent and that the polymerization process was essentially physicochemical in nature (Dorn et al 1995). More recently it has been postulated that histidine-rich proteins may form a structural focus for binding haem moieties and initiating haem polymerization in the parasite (Sullivan et al 1996). For a more detailed discussion see Ridley (1996).

Haem polymerization is inhibited by chloroquine in-vitro and probably represents the target for this drug in the parasite (Slater & Cerami 1992; Dorn et al 1995; Ridley 1996). As the process is protein independent, it was proposed that chloroquine inhibition is mediated by binding to monomeric haematin, preventing its incorporation into the growing β-haematin chain (Egan et al 1994; Dorn et al 1995). This reconciles chloroquine inhibition of haem polymerization with earlier work suggesting that haematin, or ferriprotoporphyrin IX, is the chloroquine receptor in malarial parasites (Chou et al 1980). Using isothermal titration microcalorimetry measurements it has also been demonstrated that the strength of

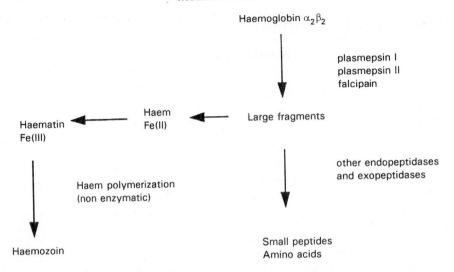

FIG. 1.   Overview of haemoglobin degradation in the acidic digestive vacuole of malaria parasites.

binding of quinoline antimalarials to haematin correlates with their ability to inhibit haem polymerization in-vitro (Dorn et al unpublished). Another consequence of the finding that haem polymerization is a physicochemical process, and that its inhibition by chloroquine does not involve interaction with parasite proteins, is that chloroquine resistance develops as a result of altered drug transport and altered drug accumulation within the parasite (Ward et al 1995). The ultimate goal of work on haem polymerization is to discover new classes of molecules that both inhibit the process of haem polymerization, and are not affected by the mutations affecting intra-parasitic drug accumulation. A high throughput haem poly-merization assay has been developed to screen chemical libraries in order to discover molecules that meet these criteria.

In addition to the screening approach, it was recently dis-covered that 4-aminoquinolines with shortened side chains, though similar in structure to chloroquine, can nevertheless overcome chloroquine resistance (Ridley et al 1996). Some examples of such compounds are shown in Table 1. It is sur-prising that compounds so closely related in structure to chloroquine manage to overcome chloroquine resistance to such a large extent. It suggests that whatever mechanisms are contributing to chloroquine resistance they are extremely structure-specific. Although promising, several aspects of these compounds require further optimization. Firstly, they retain some cross-resistance with chloroquine, i.e. they are less active against highly resistant chloroquine strains. Secondly, the desalkyl metabolites, which in the case of chloroquine con-tribute significantly to overall activity, are totally inactive against chloroquine resistant strains. Thirdly, the compounds retain similar toxic liabilities to chloroquine and this needs to be rigorously assessed.

A second class of quinoline compounds, the bisquinolines, was also shown to be active against chloroquine resistant strains (Vennerstrom et al 1992). These compounds have been investigated in some detail and the (*S*,*S*)-enantiomer of *trans*-N^1,N^2-bis(7-chloroquinolin-4-yl)cyclohexane-1,2-diamine, Ro 47-7737, was found to be particularly active against both chloroquine sensitive and chloroquine resistant strains (Fig. 2, Ridley et al 1997). The long half-life of this compound resulted

in exceptionally good curative and prophylactic activities in animal models, with a low propensity for recrudescence. Unfortunately, some toxic liabilities, especially phototoxicity, with an attendant danger of photocarcinogenicity, prevented its consideration for clinical trials.

In summary, quinoline-containing compounds still offer hope for the development of new antimalarials. However, minimalisation of toxic side-effects is essential. It should be remembered that chloroquine itself has a very low therapeutic ratio (Good & Shader 1982; Kelly et al 1990) and might have proven difficult to register in today's regulatory environment.

Inhibition of proteinases involved in haemoglobin degradation

The three proteinases studied in most detail are a cysteine proteinase, falcipain, and two aspartic proteinases, plasmepsins I and II. Because of the difficulty of working with the small quantities of enzyme available from parasite culture, the genes encoding the proteinases have been cloned and attempts made to prepare recombinant enzyme. In addition, proteinase inhi-bitors from a variety of sources have been tested for their ability to inhibit parasite growth.

The cysteine proteinase, falcipain

A cysteine proteinase activity has been identified in food vacuoles (Goldberg et al 1990; Gluzman et al 1994) and generic inhibitors of cysteine proteinases have antiparasitic effects (Rosenthal et al 1988, 1989, 1991, 1993). It is postu-lated that these inhibitors act at an early step in the hae-moglobin degradation pathway (de Gamboa & Rosenthal 1996). A cysteine proteinase gene, encoding the enzyme fal-cipain, has been cloned from most of the human malarial species (Rosenthal 1996) and it is assumed that this enzyme is responsible for the activity seen in the food vacuole extracts. However, this is not yet proven, as the food vacuole proteinase has not been purified to homogeneity for detailed molecular characterization.

There is a report that active recombinant enzyme has been successfully expressed (Salas et al 1995), but most enzyme

Table 1.   Inhibition of *P. falciparum* growth in culture by selected 4-aminoquinolines with shortened side chains.

Compound	Chain length		IC50 (nM)	
			NF54	K1
Chloroquine	n = 4		16 ± 4	315 ± 82
Ro 47-0543	n = 3		18 ± 5	59 ± 15
Ro 41-3118	n = 2		24 ± 6	49 ± 14
Ro 47-9396	n = 2		22 ± 5	50 ± 15
Ro 48-0346	n = 2		25 ± 6	61 ± 20

IC50 values are the means of a minimum of 22 independent experiments and are presented with s.d.s. The K1 strain is resistant to chloroquine and the NF54 strain is sensitive to chloroquine. Adapted from Ridley et al

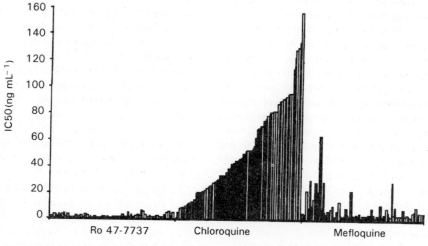

FIG. 2.   Activity of the bisquinoline Ro 47-7737, compared with chloroquine and mefloquine, against over 70 strains of *P. falciparum* malaria grown in culture. Growth was monitored over a 72-h period.

inhibitor studies rely so far on an assay involving hydrolysis of a fluorogenic substrate using malarial cell extracts (Rosenthal et al 1989). The homology of the enzyme's primary amino acid sequence to cysteine proteinases of known structure has allowed molecular models to be developed, and these models have been used to design inhibitors (Ring et al 1993). Based on modelling, it was also claimed that some chalcones with antimalarial activity worked through inhibition of cysteine proteinases, but no enzyme inhibitory data was given to confirm this (Li et al 1995). Peptidic vinylsulphones are a novel class of cysteine proteinase inhibitor shown to inhibit falcipain activity and to inhibit *P. falciparum* in culture (Rosenthal et al 1996). It was claimed that these compounds were non-toxic following oral application daily for four weeks at 30 mg kg^{-1}, but no in-vivo efficacy data was shown to demonstrate how this value compares with therapeutic doses and no pharmacokinetic evidence was given that the peptidic compounds were absorbed. The relevance of this claim is therefore unclear.

In summary, classical cysteine proteinase inhibitors inhibit parasite growth in culture, confirming falcipain as a target. Several new classes of inhibitors show activity in culture, but no specificity against human enzymes has yet been demonstrated for these compounds and no in-vivo activity has been reported.

The aspartic proteinases, plasmepsins I and II

The first aspartic proteinase to be definitively localised to the digestive vacuole of *P. falciparum* was plasmepsin I (Goldberg et al 1991). It was postulated that this enzyme initiated the process of haemoglobin degradation by cleaving the Phe$_{33}$-Leu$_{34}$ bond of the α-chain of haemoglobin. The enzyme was purified, the N-terminal sequence obtained and the gene cloned (Francis et al 1994). It initially proved difficult to express functional recombinant enzyme (Luker et al 1996) and this has only recently been achieved (Moon et al 1997).

More rapid progress at the molecular level was made with a second aspartic proteinase, plasmepsin II. The gene encoding this enzyme was first identified as part of a genomic sequencing project (Dame et al 1994) and was later successfully expressed in an active form (Hill et al 1994). In the meantime it was confirmed that this proteinase was also present in food vacuoles and that it had a substrate preference for denatured haemoglobin over native haemoglobin (Gluzman et al 1994). The recombinant enzyme has been crystallised and an X-ray structure determined (Silva et al 1996).

It is unclear why there should be two aspartic proteinases in the food vacuole. However, the availability of recombinant plasmepsin I (Moon et al 1997) now allows the specificity of the two enzymes to be assessed in detail. The distinct kinetic parameters obtained for plasmepsin I and plasmepsin II using peptide substrates, and their different susceptibility to some inhibitors, suggests that the enzymes may play different roles and have different specificities. This is reinforced by the fact that the gene encoding plasmepsin I is expressed in the ring stages, whereas the gene encoding plasmepsin II is expressed in the trophozoite stages (Moon et al unpublished).

Aspartic proteinases are a proven class of targets for cardiovascular diseases (renin) and for HIV infections (HIV protease) and there is a lot of information available on enzyme structure, mechanism and inhibition (Fusek & Vetvicka 1995). It was, therefore, possible to build up a structural model of *P. falciparum* plasmepsin I, based on gene sequence information, in the absence of crystals (Fig. 3). This advance information, coupled with the libraries of aspartic protease inhibitors already available, has assisted in an early search for inhibitors of plasmepsins.

A limited number of studies using plasmepsin inhibitors have been reported. An inhibitor of plasmepsin I inhibited *P.*

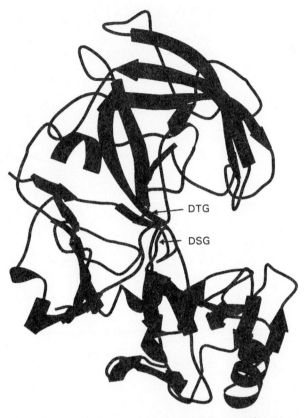

FIG. 3. Computer model of plasmepsin I, based on crystal structures of homologous aspartic proteinases. The two active-site aspartic acid (D) residues are indicated as part of their characteristic triplet (DTG and DSG) amino acid residue motifs. (This model was kindly provided by D. Bur).

falciparum growth with an IC50 of around 2 to 5 μM (Francis et al 1994) and parasite growth was inhibited at the trophozoite stage, as expected. Compounds of proven specificity for plasmepsin I have also been identified that inhibit *P. falciparum* growth at sub-micromolar levels (Moon et al 1997). A highly specific inhibitor of plasmepsin I with a K_i of 0·01 nM (compared to 1500 nM for plasmepsin II) has been reported (Luker et al 1996) but no data on the ability of this compound to inhibit parasite growth in culture was given.

With respect to plasmepsin II, an initial investigation of a limited number of inhibitors showed no striking specificities (Hill et al 1994). A compound with a 40-fold specificity of inhibition over cathepsin D ($K_i = 0·55$ nM) has been reported, but only minimal inhibition was observed against malarial parasites in culture at a concentration of 20 μM (Silva et al 1996).

In summary, the data available indicate that both plasmepsin I and plasmepsin II are valid drug targets, as inhibitors of these enzymes inhibit parasite growth in culture. Specificity against some human enzymes has been demonstrated but, like the falcipain studies, no compounds have yet been reported with in-vivo activity.

Conclusions

Inhibition of haem polymerization and the proteinases involved in haemoglobin degradation are valid approaches for the discovery of new antimalarial drugs. The challenge in the field of haem polymerization is to discover new classes of inhibitor that lack a quinoline moiety in the hope that these will both better overcome chloroquine resistance and that they will not suffer the toxic liabilities of quinolines. The challenge in the proteinase field is to convert the proteinase inhibitor activity observed in culture into an in-vivo activity in animal models and to demonstrate specificity against human enzymes. It may be that this is easier to control for the aspartic proteinase inhibitors, as the number of human aspartic proteinases is limited (Fusek & Vetvicka 1995). The availability of recombinant enzyme for high-throughput assays and crystallization studies will greatly assist these efforts.

Acknowledgements

Richard Moon, Arnulf Dorn, Colin Berry, Sudha Vippagunta and Jonathan Vennerstrom are warmly thanked for permission to quote results from unpublished manuscripts. Daniel Bur is thanked for the production of the molecular model of plasmepsin I.

References

Ball, E. G., McKee, R. W., Anfinsen, C. B., Cruz, W. O., Geumen, Q. M. (1948) Studies on malarial parasites IX. Chemical and metabolic changes during growth and multiplication in vivo and in vitro. J. Biol. Chem. 175: 547–571

Bohle, S. D., Conklin, B. J., Cox, D., Madsen, S. K., Paulson, S., Stephens, P. W., Yee, G. T. (1994) Structural and spectroscopic studies of β-hematin (the heme coordination polymer in malaria pigment). In: Wisian-Nielsen, P., Allcock, H. R., Wynne, K. J. (eds) ACS Symposium Series No. 572, Inorganic and Organometallic Polymers II: Advanced Materials and Intermediates. American Chemical Society, Columbus, Ohio, pp 497–515

Chou, A. C., Cherli, R., Fitch, C. D. (1980) Ferriprotoporphyrin IX fulfills the criteria for identification as the chloroquine receptor of malaria parasites. Biochemistry 19: 1543–1549

Dame, J. B., Reddy, G. R., Yowell, C. A., Dunn, B. M., Kay, J., Berry, C. (1994) Sequence, expression and modelled structure of an aspartic proteinase from the human malaria parasite *Plasmodium falciparum*. Mol. Biochem. Parasitol. 64: 177–190

de Gamboa, N. D., Rosenthal, P. J. (1996) Cysteine proteinase inhibitors block early steps in hemoglobin degradation by cultured malarial parasites. Blood 87: 4448–4454

Divo, A. A., Geary, T. G., Davis, N. L., Jensen, J. B. (1985) Nutritional requirements of *Plasmodium falciparum* in culture. I. Exogenously supplied dialyzable components necessary for continuous growth. J Protozool 32: 59–64

Dorn, A., Stoffel, R., Matile, H., Bubendorf, A., Ridley, R. G. (1995) Malarial haemozoin/β-haematin supports haem polymerization in the absence of protein. Nature 374: 269–271

Egan, T. J., Ross, D. C., Adams, P. A. (1994) Quinoline anti-malarial drugs inhibit spontaneous formation of β-haematin (malaria pigment). FEBS Lett. 352: 54–57

Fitch, C. D., Chevli, R., Banyal, H. S., Phillips, G., Pfaller, M. A., Krogstad, D. J. (1982) Lysis of *Plasmodium falciparum* by ferriprotoporphyrin IX and a chloroquine-ferriprotoporphyrin IX complex. Antimicrob. Agents Chemother. 21: 819–822

Fitch, C. D., Chevli, R., Kanjananggulpan, P., Dutta, P., Chevli, K., Chou, A. C. (1983) Intracellular ferriprotoporphyrin IX is a lytic agent. Blood 62: 1165–1168

Francis, S. E., Gluzman, I. Y., Oksman, A., Knickerbocker, A., Mueller, R., Bryant, M. L., Sherman, D. R., Russell, D. G., Goldberg, D. E. (1994) Molecular characterization and inhibition of a *Plasmodium falciparum* aspartic hemoglobinase. EMBO J. 13: 306–317

Fusek, M., Vetvicka, V. (1995) Aspartic Proteinases: Physiology and Pathology. CRC Press Inc., Boca Raton, Florida

Gluzman, I. Y., Francis, S. E., Oksman, A., Smith, C. E., Duffin, K. L, Goldberg, D. E. (1994) Order and specificity of the *Plasmodium*

falciparum hemoglobin degradation pathway. J. Clin. Invest. 93: 1602–1608

Goldberg, D. E., Slater, A. F. G., Cerami, A., Henderson, G. B. (1990) Hemoglobin degradation in the malaria parasite *Plasmodium falciparum*: an ordered process in a unique organelle. Proc. Natl Acad. Sci. USA 87: 2931–2935

Goldberg, D. E., Slater, A. F. G., Beavis, R., Chait, B., Cerami, A., Henderson, G. B. (1991) Hemoglobin degradation in the human malaria pathogen *Plasmodium falciparum*: a catabolic pathway initiated by a specific aspartic protease. J. Exp. Med. 173: 961–969

Good, M. I, Shader, R. I. (1982) Lethality and behavioural side effects of chloroquine. J. Clin. Psychopharmacol. 2: 40–47

Groman, N. B. (1951) Dynamic aspects of the nitrogen metabolism of *Plasmodium gallinaceum in vivo* and *in vitro*. J. Infect. Dis. 88: 126–150

Haynes, R. K., Vonwiller, S. C. (1996) The behaviour of qinghaosu (artemisinin) in the presence of heme iron (II) and (III). Tetrahedron Lett. 37: 253–256

Hill, J., Tyas, L., Phylip, L. H., Kay, J., Dunn, B. M., Berry, C. (1994) High level expression and characterisation of Plasmepsin II, an aspartic proteinase from *Plasmodium falciparum*. FEBS Lett. 352: 155–158

Kelly, J. C., Wasserman, G. S., Bernard, W. D. , Schulz, C., Knapp, J. F. (1990) Chloroquine poisoning in a child. Ann. Emerg. Med. 19: 47–50

Li, R., Kenyon, G. L., Cohen, F. E., Chen, X., Gong, B., Dominguez, J. N., Davidson, E., Kurzban, G., Miller, R. E., Nuzum, E. O. Rosenthal, P. J., McKerrow , J. H. (1995) In vitro antimalarial activity of chalcones and their derivatives. J Med Chem 38: 5031–5037

Luker, K. E., Francis, S. E., Gluzman, I. Y., Goldberg, D. E. (1996) Kinetic analysis of plasmepsins I and II, aspartic proteases of the *Plasmodium falciparum* digestive vacuole. Mol. Biochem. Parasitol. 79: 71–78

Meshnick, S. R., Taylor, T. E., Kamchonwongpaisan, S. (1996) Artemisinin and the antimalarial endoperoxides: from herbal remedy to targeted chemotherapy. Microbiol. Rev. 60: 301–315

Moon, R. P., Tyas, L., Certa, U., Rupp, K., Bur, D., Jaquet, C., Matile, H., Loetscher, H., Grueninger-Leitch, F., Kay, J., Dunn, B. M., Berry, C., Ridley, R. G. (1997) Expression and characterisation of plasmepsin I from *Plasmodium falciparum*. Eur. J. Biochem. In Press

Olliaro, P. L., Goldberg, D. E. (1995) The plasmodium digestive vacuole: Metabolic headquarters and choice drug target. Parasitol. Today 11: 294–297

Posner, G. H. (1997) Antimalarial endoperoxides that are potent and easily synthesized. J. Pharm. Pharmacol. 49 (Suppl. 2): 55–57

Rangachari, K., Dluzewski, A. R., Wilson, R. J., Gratzer, W. B. (1987) Cytoplasmic factor required for entry of malaria parasites into RBCs. Blood 70: 77–82

Ridley, R. G. (1996) Haemozoin formation in malaria parasites: is there a haem polymerase? Trends Microbiol. 4: 253–254

Ridley, R. G., Hofheinz, W., Matile, H., Jaquet, C., Dorn, A., Masciadri, R., Jolidon, S., Richter, W. F., Guenzi, A., Girometta, M.-A., Urwyler, H., Huber, W., Thaithong, S., Peters, W. (1996) 4-Aminoquinoline analogs of chloroquine with shortened side chains retain activity against chloroquine-resistant *Plasmodium falciparum*. Antimicrob. Agents Chemother. 40: 1846–1854

Ridley, R. G., Matile, H., Jaquet, C., Dorn, A., Hofheinz, W., Leupin, W., Masciadri, R., Theil, F.-P., Richter, W. F., Girometta, M.-A., Guenzi, A., Urwyler, H., Gocke, E., Potthast, J.-M., Csato, M., Thomas, A., Peters, W. (1997) Antimalarial activity of the bisquinoline $trans\text{-}N^1,N^2$-bis(7-chloroquinolin-4-yl)cyclohexane-1,2-diamine. A comparison of two stereoisomers and a detailed evaluation of the (S,S)-enantiomer, Ro 47-7737. Antimicrob. Agents Chemother. In Press

Ring, C. S., Sun, E., McKerrow, J. H., Lee, G. K., Rosenthal, P.J., Kuntz, I. D., Cohen, F. E. (1993) Structure-based inhibitor design by using protein models for the development of antiparasitic agents. Proc. Natl Acad. Sci. USA 90: 3583–3587

Rosenthal, P. J. (1996) Conservation of key amino acids among the cysteine proteinases of multiple malarial species. Mol. Biochem. Parasitol. 75: 255–260

Rosenthal, P. J., McKerrow, J. H., Aikawa, M., Nagasawa, H., Leech, J. H. (1988) A malarial cysteine proteinase is necessary for hemoglobin degradation by *Plasmodium falciparum*. J. Clin. Invest. 82: 1560–1566

Rosenthal, P. J., McKerrow, J. H., Rasnick, D., Leech, J. H. (1989) Inhibitors of lysosomal cysteine proteinases inhibit a trophozoite proteinase and block parasite development. Mol. Biochem. Parasitol. 35: 177–184

Rosenthal, P. J., Wollish, W. S., Palmer, J. T., Rasnick, D. (1991) Antimalarial effects of peptide inhibitors of a *Plasmodium falciparum* cysteine proteinase. J. Clin. Invest. 88: 1467–1472

Rosenthal, P. J., Lee, G. K., Smith, R. E. (1993) Inhibition of a *Plasmodium vinckei* cysteine proteinase cures murine malaria. J. Clin. Invest. 91: 1052–1056

Rosenthal, P. J., Olsen, J. E., Lee, G. K., Palmer, J. T., Klaus, J. L., Rasnick, D. (1996) Antimalarial effects of vinyl sulfone cysteine proteinase inhibitors. Antimicrob. Agents Chemother. 40: 1600–1603

Roth Jr., E. F., Brotman, D. S., Vanderberg, J. P., Schulman, S. (1986) Malarial pigment error in the estimation of hemoglobin content in *Plasmodium falciparum* in infected red cells: implications for metabolic and biochemical studies of the erythrocytic phases of malaria. Am. J. Trop. Med. Hyg. 35: 906–911

Salas, F., Fichmann, J., Lee, G. K., Scott, M. D., Rosenthal, P. J. (1995) Functional expression of falcipain, a *Plasmodium falciparum* cysteine proteinase, supports its role as a malarial hemoglobinase. Infect. Immun. 63: 2120–2125

Schacter, B. A. (1988) Heme catabolism by heme oxygenase: physiology, regulation and mechanism of action. Sem. Hematol. 25: 349–369

Silva, A. M., Lee, A. Y., Gulnik, S. V., Maier, P., Collins, J., Bhat, T. N., Collins, P. J., Cacheu, R. E., Luker, K., Gluzman, I. Y., Francis, S. E., Oksman, A., Goldberg, D. E., Erickson, J. W. (1996) Structure and inhibition of plasmepsin II, a haemoglobin-degrading enzyme from *Plasmodium falciaprum*. Proc. Natl Acad. Sci. USA 93: 10034–10039

Slater, A. F. G., Cerami, A. (1992) Inhibition by chloroquine of a novel haem polymerase enzyme activity in malaria trophozoites. Nature 355: 167–169

Slater, A. F. G., Swiggard, W. J., Orton, B. R., Flitter, W. D., Goldberg, D. E., Cerami, A., Henderson, G. B. (1991) An iron-carboxylate bond links the heme units of malaria pigment. Proc. Natl Acad. Sci. USA 88: 325–329

Sullivan Jr., D. J., Gluzman, I. Y., Goldberg, D. E. (1996) *Plasmodium* hemozoin formation mediated by histidine-rich proteins. Science 271: 219–222

Vander Jagt, D. L., Hunsaker, L. A., Campos, N. M., Scaletti, J. V. (1992) Localization and characterization of hemoglobin-degrading aspartic proteinases from the malarial parasite *Plasmodium falciparum*. Biochim. Biophys. Acta 1122: 256–264

Vennerstrom, J. L., Ellis, W. Y., Ager Jr., A. L., Andersen, S. L., Gerena, L., Milhous, W. K. (1992) Bisquinolines. 1. *N,N*-Bis(7-chloroquinolin-4yl)alkanediamines with potential against chloroquine-resistant malaria. J. Med. Chem. 35: 2129–2134

Ward, S. A., Bray, P. G., Mungthin, M., Hawley, S. R. (1995) Current views on the mechanisms of resistance to quinoline-containing drugs in *Plasmodium falciparum*. Ann. Trop. Med. Parasitol. 89: 121–124

Zarchin, S., Krugliak, M., Ginsburg, H. (1986) Digestion of the host erythrocyte by malaria parasites is the primary target for quinoline-containing antimalarials. Biochem. Pharmacol. 35: 2435–2442

J. Pharm. Pharmacol. 1997, 49 (Suppl. 2): 49–53

Haem-mediated Decomposition of Artemisinin and its Derivatives: Pharmacological and Toxicological Considerations

GEOFFREY EDWARDS

Department of Pharmacology and Therapeutics, The University of Liverpool and Division of Parasite and Vector Biology, Liverpool School of Tropical Medicine

Resistance of *Plasmodium falciparum* to currently available antimalarial drugs is intensifying the search for novel, more effective chemotherapeutic agents. The most important discovery, isolated by Chinese scientists from *Artemisia annua*, is artemisinin (Klayman 1985; Meshnick et al 1996; Fig. 1). Despite impressive biological activity, problems with recrudescence and difficulties with formulation have led to the development of artemether and arteether. These are methyl and ethyl ethers of dihydroartemisinin, a lactone-reduced analogue of artemisinin and are more potent than artemisinin in-vitro and in-vivo in animal studies. Water soluble derivatives of dihydroartemisinin, artesunate and sodium artelinate have also been produced (Fig. 2). These analogues are at various stages of development. Artemether and sodium artesunate are in clinical use and are under evaluation in multi-centre trials (Hien & White 1993), arteether is being developed jointly by the World Health Organization (WHO) and the Walter Reed Army Institute of Research and sodium artelinate is in phase I clinical trials (Olliaro & Trigg 1995). Clinical studies worldwide with artemisinin and its analogues have shown these drugs to be particularly effective in the treatment of severe malaria and in cases of *Plasmodium falciparum* infection unresponsive to treatment with existing antimalarial agents (White 1994; Li et al 1994; Hien 1994; Looareesuwan 1994; Salako et al 1994). Their efficacy and relatively low clinical toxicity has encouraged their widespread and occasionally unregulated use. A concern was raised, not unreasonably, that these drugs were being used against a background of pharmacological ignorance as, aside from the Chinese literature, there was relatively little definitive information on the pharmacology of these substances. Information was circulating within internal documents of the US Army and the WHO but not in peer-reviewed journals generally available to Western scientists. A major stimulus to activity in this area was provided by a meeting organized under the auspices of the Wellcome Trust in April 1993. At this meeting, a group of scientists and clinicians active in this field met to exchange views. While the success of artemisinin and its analogues was acknowledged, several gaps in our knowledge became apparent, notably the empirical nature of dosage regimens for these drugs and the evidence of neurotoxicity in preclinical studies.

Pharmacology

There was, until recently, relatively little published pharmacokinetic information on artemisinin in Western literature

Correspondence: G. Edwards, Department of Pharmacology and Therapeutics, The University of Liverpool, Liverpool L69 3BX, UK. E-Mail: ge1000@liv.ac.uk

(Titulaer et al 1990) but a proliferation of activity in this area leads us to hope that rationally-derived dosage regimens might not be too far away (Duc et al 1994; Na Bangchang et al 1994; Hassan Alin et al 1996a, b). However, much of the available information is descriptive, and the relationship between pharmacokinetics and drug response is poorly understood. The principal drawback to acquiring such information is that the development of analytical methodology for measurement of

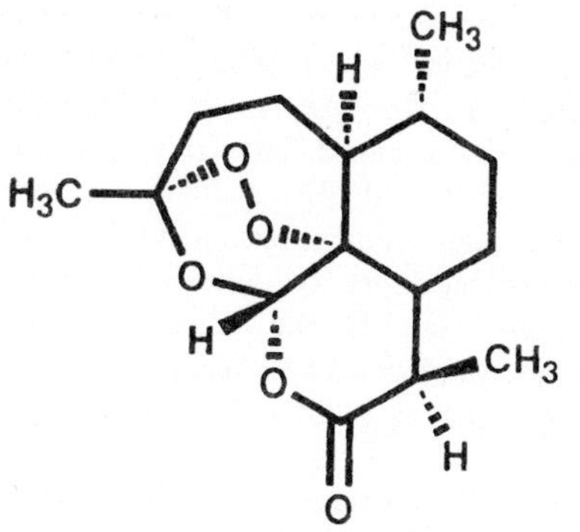

FIG. 1. Chemical structure of artemisinin.

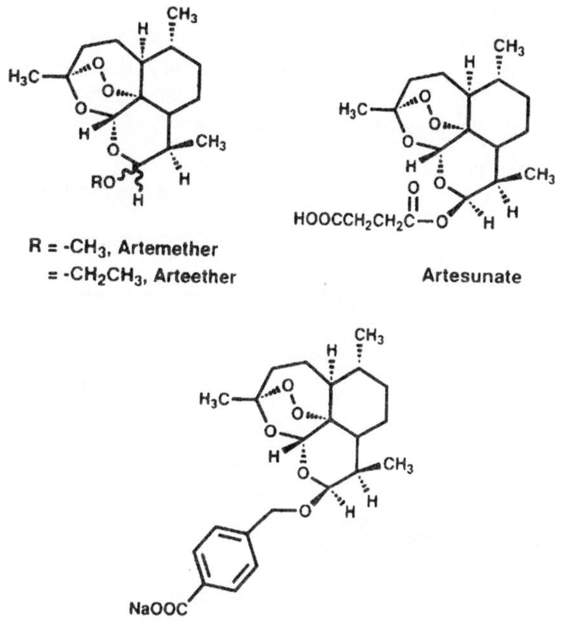

R = -CH₃, Artemether
= -CH₂CH₃, Arteether

Artesunate

Sodium artelinate

FIG. 2. Chemical structures of artemether, arteether, artesunate and sodium artelinate.

these agents in biological fluids poses challenging problems (Edwards 1994). There has also been concern about what should be measured and whether these measurements are accurate markers of biological activity (Edwards et al 1992). Two main approaches to analysis have been adopted. These have each used high-performance liquid chromatography (HPLC) with either electrochemical (EC) (Melendez et al 1991) or ultra-violet (UV) detection. None of the derivatives of artemisinin possesses a suitable chromophore, so pre- (Idowu et al 1989; Thomas et al 1992; Muhia et al 1994a or post-column (Edlund et al 1984; Batty et al 1996) derivatization has been used. While evaluating a method for the measurement of artemether in whole blood, it became clear that there were significant losses of this analyte in samples stored under different conditions. This suggests decomposition of artemether, sequestration within or binding to the erythrocytic membrane (Edwards et al 1992). Furthermore, work from Meshnick and co-workers pointed to the formation of an adduct of artemisinin and haem and ferriprotoporphyrin-catalysed decomposition of artemisinin and its analogues (Meshnick et al 1991; Hong et al 1994). Several lines of evidence point to the peroxide linkage, a common feature of the molecular structure of artemisinin and its analogues, playing a major role in these phenomena (Fig. 3). The chemistry of the haem-artemisinin interaction has been explored thoroughly by Posner and his colleagues (Cumming et al 1996) and will be reviewed in this issue. Our studies have demonstrated that two major products, probably hydroxylated desoxy derivatives, arise from the reaction of haemin in-vitro with radioactively labelled artemether. The rate and extent of formation of these species are time dependent and are enhanced by increasing the concentration of haemin. We have shown also that erythrocyte haemolysis products accelerate the decomposition of artemether (Muhia et al 1994b). In plasma samples from patients with malaria, breakdown products of haemoglobin may be present in sufficient quantities to facilitate the decomposition of artemisinin derivatives. All of this causes concern when attempting to relate drug concentrations to a pharmacological response or when building in blood clearance to a pharmacokinetic model. Since the stimulus for pharmacological effect is the unbound drug concentation, binding to blood cells should

not pose a major difficulty. However, problems could arise if the rate of disappearance of artemisinin and its analogues from blood is relatively rapid compared with total blood clearance.

Neurotoxicity

There is some concern that the use of artemisinin and its analogues against a background of limited pharmacological information, despite wide clinical experience, could yield some unexpected observations. As if to emphasize this point, a series of in-vivo toxicity studies in the dog and rat, injected intramuscularly with artemether and arteether, revealed a dose-dependent neurotoxicity associated with movement disturbances and spasticity. The neuropathies were specific to the caudal brain stem and were characterized by swollen axonal processes and spheroid formation with associated axonal degredation and necrosis in myelinated axons (Brewer et al 1994a,b). Furthermore, studies in monkeys (*Macacca mulatta*) demonstrated a dose-dependent neuropathology in the same regions as rodent and canine brains (Petras et al 1994). These histological changes have been found in the absence of neurological signs or behavioural performance deficits (Genovese et al 1995). Recent observations in-vitro from this laboratory (Fishwick et al 1994) and the Walter Reed Army Institute of Research in the USA (Wesche et al 1994) have shown inhibition of neuronal cell proliferation. It may be argued that this is a manifestation of general cytotoxicity as other cell types, such as Ehrlich ascites tumour cells (Woerdenbag et al 1993) and 3T3 kidney fibroblasts have been shown to be susceptible to artemisinin, albeit at higher concentrations. It is therefore more relevant to examine in-vitro the effects of these agents under conditions more reflective of axonal growth and maintenance in-vivo. When cultured in medium lacking serum but containing dibutyryl cyclic AMP, Nb2a cells differentiate and project extensions or neurites that are branching varicose processes similar to those produced by sympathetic neurones in primary cell culture (Prasad & Hsie 1971). In addition, there is expression of a variety of neuronal proteins including growth-associated polypeptide GAP-43, the neurofilament triplet proteins and the enzyme ornithine decarboxylase (Abdulla & Campbell 1993). These neuronal properties are affected by a

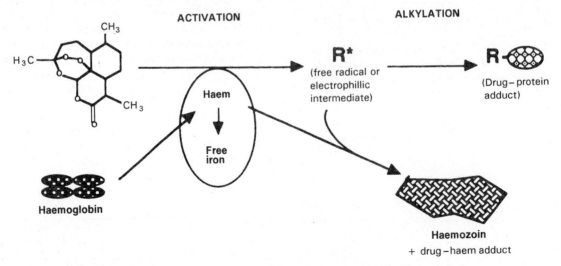

FIG. 3.   Activation of artemisinin and its reaction with haem and proteins (from Meshnick 1994, with permission).

wide range of toxic agents and are subject to alteration in neuropathies. Therefore, Nb2a cells provide a good model for studying the effects of neurotoxins on nerve outgrowth in develooment and regeneration, and also the integrity of the axonal cytoskeleton.

Looking at the effects of artemisinin, its derivatives and metabolites on the production of neurites in mouse neuroblastoma Nb2a cells, dihydroartemisinin was the most inhibitory. Recent findings from our laboratory have identified an IC50 value for dihydroartemisinin of approximately 0.35 μM. Other derivatives and analogues appear less toxic (Fishwick et al 1995). Such effects on neurite outgrowth occur at concentrations significantly less than those needed to reduce cellular proliferation and suggest some degree of specificity for neuronal cells. Proliferating neuroblastoma cells do not express the phenotypes of cells in the mature nervous system, for instance they do not possess axons or dendrites and effects on proliferation may not reflect selective neurotoxicity.

Clearly, if dihydroartemisinin crosses the blood–brain barrier to give concentrations in cerebrospinal fluid equivalent to those in serum (ca. 2.5 μM) then brain-stem toxicity might arise (Wesche et al 1994). However, much depends on the rate and route of administration and the relative conversion of the administered derivative to dihydroartemisinin as evidenced by the absence of reports of neurotoxicity in any clinical study (Phillips-Howard & ter Kuile 1995). Since these agents are used mostly in severely ill or comatose patients in whom there may be disease-related nerological sequelae, it may be impossible to identify drug-induced neurotoxicity in a clinical environment.

Enhancement of neurotoxicity by ferriprotoporphyrin

With a body of evidence pointing to a central role for ferriprotoporphyrin in the pharmacological actions of artemisinin, its derivatives and analogues, it is of interest to know whether their neurotoxicity is enhanced by haem. Using two methods of assessment, the metabolism of the tetrazolium salt 3-(4,5 diethylthiazol-2-yl)-2,5-diphenyl-tetrazolium bromide (MTT) or the inhibition of neurite outgrowth, haemin potentiates the neurotoxicity of artemether, arteether or dihydroartemisinin in a dose-dependent fashion without an effect by itself (Smith et al 1996) . Haemin also increases the concentration-related binding of radiolabelled (^{14}C) dihydroartemisinin to proteins from Nb2a cells two-fold and to rat brain three- to six-fold (Fishwick et al 1996). It has already been reported that antimarial endoperoxides react with specific proteins in the malarial parasite *Plasmodium falciparum* under physiological conditions (Asawamahasakda et al 1994) and that in haemoproteins, haem catalyses the alkylation of the protein moiety (Yang et al 1994). Haemin does not enhance the neurotoxicity of desoxyarteether, a structural analogue of arteether without an endoperoxide bridge (Smith et al 1996) and this analogue does not interact covalently with serum albumin (Yang et al 1993, 1994). These findings suggest the mechanism of neurotoxicity is similar to the mechanism of antimalarial activity. It is probable that haemin is catalysing the decomposition of artemisinin and its analogues to reactive species (Zhang et al 1992; Meshnick et al 1993) that are toxic to neuronal cells. Ferriprotoporphyrin (and free iron) can accelerate the decomposition of artemisinin and its derivatives through cleavage of the endoperoxide bridge to produce a carbon-centred radical (Posner & Oh 1992; Posner et al 1994, 1995a) possibly via an iron-oxo intermediate (Posner et al 1995b). It is unlikely that free iron, released from haemin during a reaction with artemisinin derivatives, is responsible for the neurotoxic effects as Fe^{2+} (ferrous sulphate) fails to enhance the toxicity of dihydroartemisinin in rat neurobastoma X glioma hybrid cells (Parker et al 1994). Damage may occur by lipid peroxidation or protein oxidation in neuronal membranes or cytoskeleton. Artesunate produces lipid peroxidation and oxidises thiol groups in isolated erythrocytic membranes (Meshnick et al 1989, 1991). Interestingly, one of the products of the iron-catalysed cleavage of endoperoxides like artemisinin, is a 1,5 diketone (Posner et al 1995a,b, 1996), a potent alkylating agent. This may crosslink cytoskeletal proteins in a fashion analogous to hexacarbon diketones such as 2,5 hexanedione (Genter St Clair et al 1988). Artemisinin binds to actin and, interestingly, the haem-containing protein spectrin, which is related closely to fodrin, a protein involved in cytosleletal maintenance (Asawamahasakda et al 1994; Lai & Singh 1995).

Conclusions

The isolation by Chinese scientists of artemisinin and the development of its derivatives can be considered to represent the most important breakthrough in malaria chemotherapy in recent times. Our increased understanding of the pharmacology of these agents allows the development of novel compounds of greater potency (Posner 1997). Moreover their unique mechanism of action should permit their use to continue with minimal interruption from the spectre of drug resistance that has dogged malaria chemotherapy with conventional chemotherapeutic agents. However, caution must be exercized and indiscriminate prophylactic usage could prove problematic. For severe malaria, it is vital that their use is rationalised and the role of sub-optimal therapy in the observed recrudescence be addressed. To do this, analytical methodology must be valid and appropriate. The question of whether preclinical neurotoxicity is an important clinical consideration remains uncertain, as no study has yet been designed to address this issue. Evidence from in-vitro investigations points to dihydroartemisinin, a common metabolite of artemether, arteether and artesunate, as being particularly neurotoxic, although rate and route of administration of the drug in question is important. Early evidence points to the half-life of dihydroartemisinin derived from intravenous artesunate being relatively short (Batty et al 1996). Alternatively, the benefit that these drugs undoubtedly convey in the treatment of severe disease may outweigh any theoretical risk of toxicity (Nosten & Price 1995). Importantly, neurological sequelae of cerebral malaria may not be distinguishable from drug-related effects. However, we should realise that we are dealing with chemicals that are organic peroxides of dubious stability and should be aware of unforeseen effects that might arise from their uncontrolled application.

Acknowledgements
Original work by the author was supported by the Medical Research Council, the Wellcome Trust and the UNDP/WHO/ World Bank Special Programme for Research and Training in Tropical Diseases.

References

Abdulla, E. M., Campbell, I. C. (1993) Use of neurite outgrowth as an *in vitro* method of assessing neurotoxicity. Ann. NY Acad. Sci. 679: 276–279

Asawamahasakda, W., Benakis, A., Meshnick, S. R. (1994) The interaction of artemisinin with red cell membranes. J. Lab. Clin. Med. 123: 757–762

Batty, K. T., Davis, T. M. E., Thu, L. T. A., Binh, T. Q., Anh, T. K., Ilett, K. F. (1996) Selective high-performance liquid chromatographic determination of artesunate and α- and β-dihydroartemisinin in patients with falciparum malaria. J. Chromatogr. 677: 345–350

Brewer, T. G., Peggins, J. O., Grate, S. J., Petras, J. M., Levine, B. S., Weina, P. J., Swearengen, J., Heiffer, M. H., Schuster, B. G. (1994a) Neurotoxicity in animals due to arteether and artemether. Trans. R. Soc. Trop. Med. Hyg. 88 (Suppl. 1): 33–36

Brewer, T. G., Grate, S. J., Peggins, J. O., Weina, P. J., Petras, J. M., Levine, B. S., Heifer, M. H., Schuster, B. G. (1994b) Fatal neurotoxicity of arteether and artemether. Am. J. Trop. Med. Hyg. 51: 251–259

Cumming, J. R., Ploypradith, P., Posner, G. H. (1997) Antimalarial activity of artemisinin (qinghaosu) and related trioxanes: mechanism of action,. Adv. Pharmacol. 37: 253–297

Duc, D. D., De Vries, P. J., Khanh, N. X., Binh, L. N., Kager, P. A., van Boxrtel, C. J. (1994) The pharmacokinetics of a single dose of artemisinin in healthy Vietnamese subjects. Am. J. Trop. Med. Hyg. 51: 785–790

Edlund, P.O., Westerlund, D., Carlqvist, J., Bo-Liang, W., Yunhua, J. (1984) Determination of artesunate and dihydroartemisinine in plasma by liquid chromatography with post-column derivatisation and UV-detection. Acta. Pharm. Suec. 21: 223–234

Edwards, G. (1994) Measurement of artemisinin and its derivatives in biological fluids. Trans. R. Soc. Trop. Med. Hyg. 88 (Suppl. 1): 37–39

Edwards, G., Ward, S. A., Breckenridge, A. M. (1992) Interaction of arteether with the red blood cell *in vitro* and its possible importance in the interpretation of plasma concentrations in vivo. J. Pharm. Pharmacol. 44: 280–281

Fishwick, J., McLean, W. G., Edwards, G., Ward, S. A. (1995) The toxicity of artemisinin and related compounds on neuronal and glial cells in culture. Chem. Biol. Interact. 96: 263–271

Fishwick, J., McLean, W. G., Edwards, G., Ward, S. A. (1996) Investigation of the mechanism of neurotoxicity of the artemisinin derivatives. Trans. R. Soc. Trop. Med. Hyg. 90: 211

Genovese, R. F., Petras, J. M., Brewer, T. G. (1995) Arteether neurotoxicity in the absence of deficits in behavioural performance in rats. Ann. Trop. Med. Parasitol. 89: 447–449

Genter St Clair, M. B., Amaranth, V., Moody, A. M., Anthony, D. C., Anderson, C. W., Graham, D. C. (1988) Pyrrole oxidation and protein cross-linking as necessary steps in the development of γ-ketone neuropathy. Chem. Res. Toxicol. 1: 179–185

Hassan Alin, M., Ashton, M., Kihamia, C. M., Mtey, G. J. B., Bjorkman, A. (1996a) Multiple dose pharmacokinetics of oral artemisinin and comparison of its efficacy with that of oral artesunate in falciparum malaraia patients. Trans. R. Soc. Trop. Med. Hyg. 90: 61–65

Hassan Alin, M., Ashton, M., Kihamia, C. M., Mtey, G. J. B., Bjorkman, A. (1996b) Clinical efficacy and pharmacokinetics of artemisinin monotherapy and in combination with mefloquine in patients with falciparum malaria. Br. J. Clin. Pharmacol. 41: 587–592

Hien, T. T. (1994) An overview of the clinical use of artemisinin and its derivatives in the treatment of falciparum malaria in Vietnam. Trans. R. Soc. Trop. Med. Hyg. 88 (Suppl. S1): 7–8

Hien, T. T., White, N. J. (1993) Qinghaosu. Lancet 341: 603–608

Hong, Y-L., Yang, Y-Z., Meshnick, S. R. (1994) The interaction of artemisinin with malarial hemozoin. Mol. Biochem. Parasitol. 63: 121–128

Idowu, O. R., Edwards, G., Ward, S. A., Orme, M. L' E., Breckenridge, A. M. (1989) Determination of arteether in blood plasma by high-performance liquid chromatography with ultraviolet detection after hydrolysis with acid . J. Chromatogr. 493: 125–136

Klayman, D. L. (1985) Qinghaosu (artemisinin): an antimalarial drug from China. Science 228: 1049–1055

Lai, H., Singh, N. P. (1995) Selective cancer cell cytotoxicity from exposure to dihydroartemisinin and holotransferrin. Cancer Lett. 91: 41–46

Li, G-Q., Guo, X-B., Fu, L-C., Jian, H-X., Wang, X-H. (1994) Clinical trials on artemisinin and its derivatives in the treatment of malaria in China. Trans. R. Soc. Trop. Med. Hyg. 88 (Supppl. 1): 5–6

Looareesuwan, S. (1994) Overview of clinical studies on artemisinin derivatives in Thailand. Trans. R. Soc. Trop. Med Hyg. 88 (Suppl. 1): 9–11

Melendez, V., Peggins, J. O., Brewer, T. G., Theoharides, A. D. (1991) Determination of the antimalarial arteether and its deethylated metabolite dihydroartemisinin by high-performance liquid chromatography with electrochemical detection. J. Pharm. Sci. 80: 132–138

Meshnick, S. R., Tsang, T. W., Lin, F.-B., Pan, H.-Z., Chang, C.-N., Kuypers, F., Chiu, D., Lubin, B. (1989) Activated oxygen mediates the antimalarial activity of qinghaosu. Prog. Clin. Biol. Res. 313: 95–104

Meshnick, S. R., Thomas, A., Ranz, A., Xu, C.-M., Pan, H.-Z. (1991) Artemisinin (qinghaosu): the role of intracellular hemin in its mechanism of antimalarial action. Mol. Biochem. Parasitol. 49: 181–190

Meshnick, S. R., Yang, Y.-L., Lima, V., Kuypers, F., Kamchonwongpaisan, S., Yuthavong, Y. (1993) Iron dependent free-radical generation from the antimalarial agent artemisinin (qinghaosu). Antimicrob. Agents. Chemother. 37: 1108–1114

Meshnick, S. R. (1994) The mode of action of antimalarial endoperoxides. Trans. R. Soc. Trop. Med. Hyg. 88 (Suppl. 1): 31–32

Meshnick, S. R., Taylor, T. E., Kamchonwongpaisan, S. (1996) Artemisinin and the antimalarial endoperoxides: from herbal remedy to targeted chemotherapy. Microbiol. Rev. 60: 301–305

Muhia, D. K., Mberu, E. K., Watkins, W. M. (1994a) Differential extraction of artemether and its metabolite dihydroartemisinin from plasma and determination by high-performance liquid chromatography. J Chromatogr. 660: 196–199

Muhia, D. K., Thomas, C. G., Ward, S. A., Edwards, G., Mberu, E. K., Watkins, W. M. (1994b) Ferriprotoporphyrin catalysed decomposition of artemether: analytical and pharmacological implications. Biochem. Pharmacol. 48: 889–895

Na Bangchang, K., Karbwang, J., Thomas, C. G., Thanavibul, A., Sukontason, K., Ward, S. A, Edwards, G. (1994) Pharmacokinetics of artemether after oral administration to healthy Thai males and patients with acute uncomplicated falciparum malaria. Br. J. Clin. Pharmacol. 37: 249–253

Nosten, F., Price, R. N. (1995) New antimalarials. A risk benefit analysis. Drug Safety 12: 264–273

Olliaro, P., Trigg, P. I. (1995) Status of antimalarial drugs under development. Bull. Wld. Hlth. Org. 73: 565–571

Parker, F. C., Wesche, D. L., Brewer, T.G. (1994) Does iron have a role in dihydroartemisinin-induced in vitro neurotoxicity? Am. J. Trop. Med. Hyg. 51: 260 (abstract)

Petras, J. M., Kyle, D. E., Ngampochjana, M., Young, G. D., Webster, H. K., Corcoran, K. D., Peggins, J. O., Brewer, T. G. (1994) Arteether-induced brainstem injury in *Macaca mulatta*. Am. J. Trop. Med. Hyg. 51: 100 (abstract)

Phillips-Howard, P. A., ter Kuile, F. (1995) CNS adverse events associated with antimalarial agents: fact or fiction? Drug Safety 13: 370–383

Posner, G. H., Oh, C. H. (1992) A regiospecifically oxygen-18 labelled 1,2,4-trioxane: a simple chemical model system to probe the mechanism(s) for the antimalarial activity of artemisinin (qinghaosu). J. Am. Chem. Soc. 114: 8328–8329

Posner, G.H., Oh, C. H., Wang, D., Gerena, L., Milhous, W. K., Meshnick, S. R., Asawamahasakda, W. (1994) Mechanism-based design, synthesis, and in vitro testing of new 4-methylated trioxanes structurally related to artemisinin: the importance of a carbon-centered radical for antimalarial activity. J. Med. Chem. 37: 1256–1258

Posner, G. H., Wang, D., Cumming, J. N., Oh, C. H., French, A. N., Bodley, A. L., Shapiro, T. A. (1995a) Further evidence supporting the importance of and the restrictions on a carbon-centered radical for high antimalarial activity of 1,2,4-trioxanes like artemisinin. J. Med. Chem. 38: 2273–2275

Posner, G. H., Cumming, J. N., Ploypradith, P., Oh, C. H. (1995b) Evidence for Fe(IV)=O in the molecular mechanism of action of the trioxane antimalarial artemisinin. J. Am. Chem. Soc. 17: 5885–5886

Posner, G. H., Sheldon, B. P., Gonzalez, L., Wang, D., Cumming, J. N., Klinedinst, D., Shapiro, T. A., Bachi, M. D. (1996) Evidence for the importance of high valent Fe=O and of a diketone in the molecular mechanism of action of antimalarial trioxane analogs of artemisinin. J. Am. Chem. Soc. 118: 3537–3538

Posner, G. H. (1997) Antimalarial endoperoxides that are potent and easily synthesized. J. Pharm. Pharmacol. 49 (Suppl. 2): 55–57

Prasad, K. N., Hsie, A. W. (1971) Morphological differentiation of mouse neuroblastoma cells induced in vitro by dibutyryl adenosine 3'-5' cyclic monophosphate. Nature New Biol. 233: 141–142

Salako, L. A., Walker, O., Sowunmi, S. J., Omokhodion, S. J., Adio, R., Oduola, A. M. J. (1994) Artemether in moderately severe and cerebral malaria in Nigerian children. Trans. R. Soc. Trop. Med. Hyg. 88 (Suppl. 1): 13–15

Smith, S. L., McLean, W. G., Edwards, G., Ward, S. A. (1996) Haemin augements the in vitro neurotoxicity of artemisinin derivatives. Trans. R. Soc. Trop. Med. Hyg. 90: 215

Thomas, C. G., Ward, S. A., Edwards, G. (1992) The simultaneous determination, on plasma, of artemether and its major metabolite dihydroartemisinin by high-performance liquid chromatography with ultraviolet detection. J. Chromatogr. 583: 131–139

Titulaer, H. A. C., Zuidema, J., Kager, P. A., Wetseyn, J. C. F. M., Lugt, C. B., Merkus, F. W. H. M. (1990) The pharmacokinetics of artemisinin after oral, intramuscular and rectal administration to volunteers. J. Pharm. Pharmacol. 42: 810–813

Wesche, D. L., Decoster, M. A., Tortella, F. C., Brewer, T. G. (1994) Neurotoxicity of artemisinin analogs in-vitro. Antimicrob. Agents. Chemother. 38: 1813–1819

White, N. J. (1994) Artemisinin: current status. Trans. R. Soc. Trop. Med. Hyg. 88 (Suppl 1): 3–4

Woerdenbag, H. J., Moskal, T. A., Pras, N., Malingre, T. M. (1993) Cytotoxicity of artemisinin and related endoperoxides to Ehrlich ascites tumor cells. J. Nat. Prod. 56: 849–856

Yang, Y.-Z., Asawamahasakda, W., Meshnick, S. R. (1993) Alkylation of human albumin by the antimalarial artemisinin. Biochem. Pharmacol. 46: 336–339

Yang, Y.-Z., Little, B., Meshnick, S. (1994) Alkylation of proteins by artemisinin. Biochem. Pharmacol. 48: 569–573

Zhang, F., Gosser, D. K., Meshnick, S. R. (1992) Hemin-catalysed decomposition of artemisinin (qinghaosu). Biochem. Pharmacol. 43: 1805–1809

J. Pharm. Pharmacol. 1997, 49 (Suppl. 2): 55–57

Antimalarial Endoperoxides that are Potent and Easily Synthesized

GARY H. POSNER

Department of Chemistry, Johns Hopkins University, Baltimore, MD 21218, USA

The rapidly increasing resistance of *Plasmodium falciparum* malaria parasites to previously efficacious alkaloidal drugs like chloroquine has prompted a worldwide search for new classes of compounds, not only for malaria chemoprophylaxis but also for chemotherapy, especially of acute malaria (Cumming et al 1996; Meshnick et al 1996). This search has led to the development of the fluorinated alkaloid drugs mefloquine (Sweeney 1981) and halofantrine (Goldsmith 1992) and also to the isolation and characterization of the potent and fast-acting 1,2,4-trioxane artemisinin (qinghaosu, 1) (Fig. 1), as the active antimalarial component of a plant extract used in China for over two thousand years as a herbal remedy for malaria (Zhou & Xu 1994). Also, this search has recently led to much structure-activity relationship study of 1,2,4-trioxanes (Avery et al 1996) and to an understanding of the fundamental biological (Meshnick et al 1996) and chemical (Cumming et al 1996) mechanisms of actions of such trioxanes.

Malaria parasites self-destruct after encountering a trioxane (Meshnick et al 1996). Triggered by the iron-rich environment inside the malaria parasite, the trioxane is chemically reduced by ferrous ions. This process ruptures the peroxidic oxygen-oxygen bond of the trioxane and forms an oxygen-centered free radical (a reactive oxygen species). Being a reactive intermediate, this oxygen radical can undergo various subsequent chemical transformations. One such transformation that is important for high antimalarial activity is a 1,5-hydrogen atom shift to form a somewhat more stable carbon-centered free radical intermediate (Fig. 2) (Posner et al 1994).

Immediately thereafter, the carbon radical fragments to release a stable organic vinylic ether and a reactive high-valent iron-oxo intermediate (Posner et al 1995). Evidence for this high energy iron-oxo species rests on several different kinds of trapping experiments. This iron-oxo species itself can kill the malaria parasite by oxygenating and thereby disrupting various vital biomolecules inside the parasite, and/or the iron-oxo species can epoxidize the vinylic ether to form an alkylating and therefore damaging epoxide (Fig. 2).

Based on this understanding at the molecular level of the chemical mechanism of artemisinin's antimalarial activity, a

structural and synthetically much simpler class of peroxides has been developed. These endoperoxides (not trioxanes) were designed as inexpensive and easily synthesized (two steps from commercial reactants) compounds that were expected to kill malaria parasites (Fig. 3) (Posner et al 1996a). Phenyl endoperoxide **2a**, prepared on a multigram scale, is a crystalline solid that is stable, even at 60°C, for at least 24 h. It does indeed kill malaria parasites; on a nanomolar basis, endoperoxide **2a** has about 12% of the in-vitro antimalarial activity of the complex sequiterpene natural product artemisinin (**1**). Thus, this initial success is proof that the concept is valid;

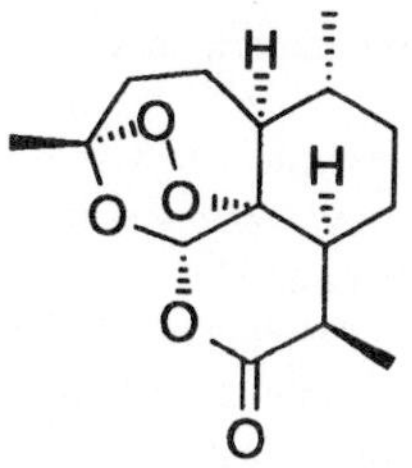

FIG. 1. Chemical structure of artemesinin (qinghaosu).

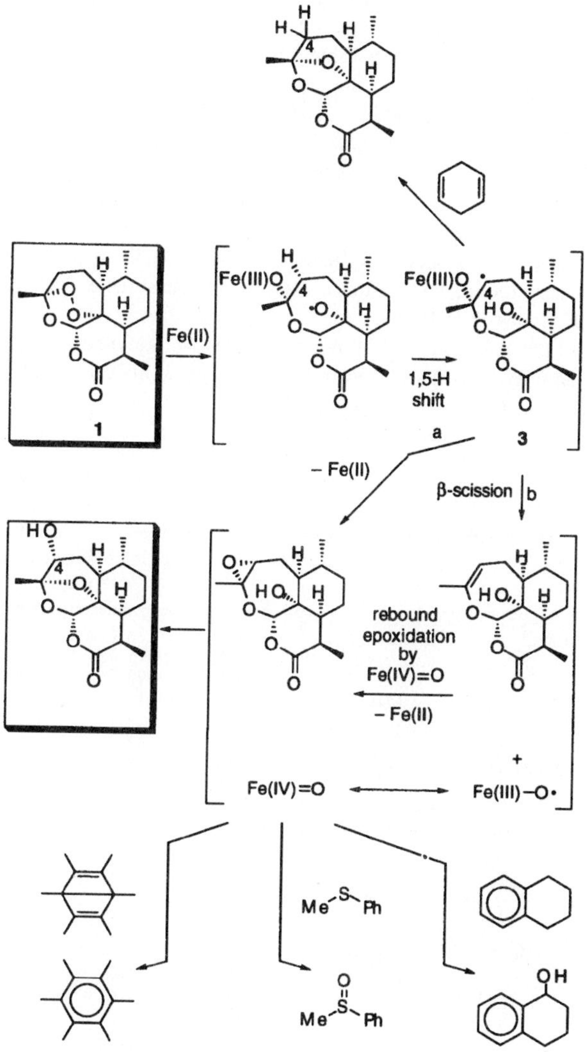

FIG. 2. Mechanism of artemisinin's reduction by iron (II).

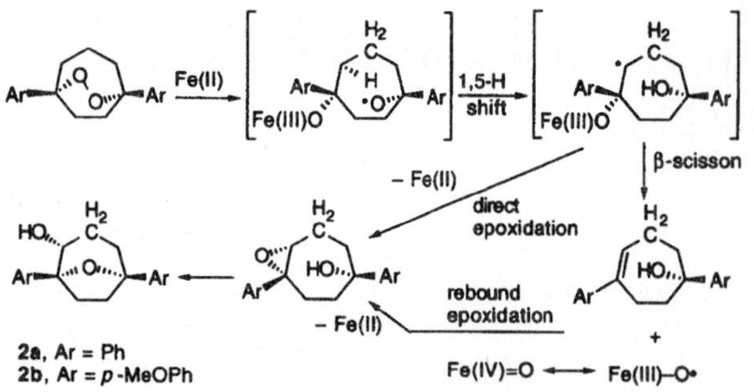

FIG. 3. Synthesis of diaryl bicyclic [3.2.2.] endoperoxides.

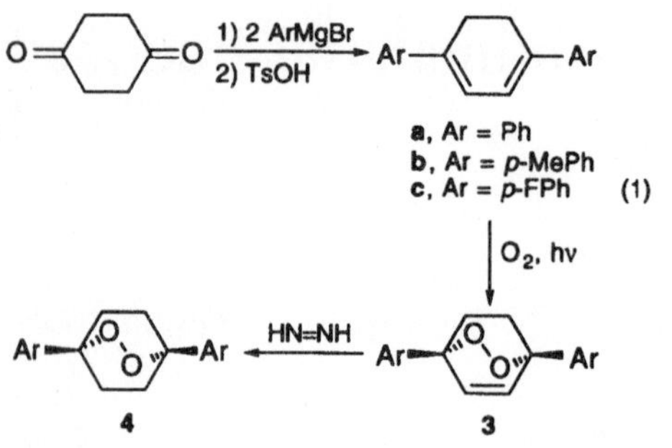

FIG. 4. Synthesis of diaryl bicyclic [2.2.2.] endoperoxides.

some mechanistically designed, structurally simple, and easily synthesized endoperoxides are indeed antimalarial, and therefore further study to prepare analogs with optimized potency and minimized possible toxicity is clearly worthwhile.

As an initial exploration of its possible toxicity and its possible activity against other parasites, endoperoxide 2a was examined further. Because humans with compromised immune systems are susceptible to *Toxoplasma gondii* parasites that often cause opportunistic infections such as cerebral encephalitis (Ou-Yang et al 1990), endoperoxide 2a was examined in-vitro for its activity against *T. gondii* in cultured L929 cells; the results are shown in Table 1 in comparison with the drugs atovaquone and artemisinin (1).

At 1.0-µM concentrations, endoperoxide 2a is approximately comparable to artemisinin in potency. What is especially promising is the therapeutic index (activity/toxicity ratio) characteristic of endoperoxide 2a at 1.0-µM concentration (Table 1): atovaquone, 95.2 / 17.4 = 5.5; artemisinin, 75.8 / 10.3 = 7.4; endoperoxide 2a, 69.6/0 = ≫ 100. Even at 10-µM concentration, endoperoxide 2a has no measurable toxicity (Fishwick et al 1995).

Like bicyclic [3·2·2] endoperoxide 2a, bicyclic [2·2·2] endoperoxides 3 and 4 were prepared very easily and rapidly (Fig. 4) (Posner et al 1996b).

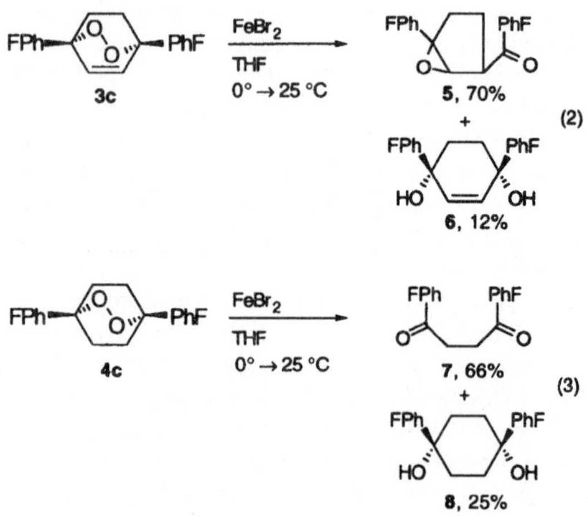

FIG. 5. Reduction of fluorophenyl endoperoxides.

Although the phenyl and the tolyl endoperoxides 3a, 3b, and 4a are not very potent antimalarials, both the unsaturated *p*-fluorophenyl endoperoxide 3c and the saturated *p*-fluorophenyl endoperoxide 4c have, on a nanomolar basis, approximately 15% of the antimalarial activity of the structurally complex, natural, clinically used, trioxane artemisinin (1). Both inexpensive and easily accessible fluorophenyl endoperoxides 3c and 4c are crystalline compounds, stable for at least 40 h at 60°C (Posner et al 1996b). In the presence of ferrous bromide, both fluorinated endoperoxides 3c and 4c are reduced rapidly to form products 5–8 (Fig. 5). A plausible mechanism to account for these FeBr₂ reductions is depicted in Fig. 6. Reductive cleavage of the weak peroxide bond followed, in pathway a, by a second electron transfer from iron(II) and liberation of two equivalents of Fe(III) produces 1,4-diols 6 and 8. Carbonyl formation, as in pathway b, releases a carbon-centered radical that fragments to form ethylene and the observed 1,4-diketone 7; alternatively via pathway b, the unsaturated carbon radical cyclizes and directly forms the observed epoxy cyclopentane ketone 5 as a single diastereomer.

Although reduction products 6–8 showed virtually no in-vitro antimalarial activity when tested as pure compounds, epoxy ketone 5 has measurable antimalarial activity. Thus, unsaturated fluorophenyl endoperoxide 3c may be a prodrug triggered by iron(II), inside a malaria parasite, to release electrophilic epoxy ketone 5 that itself or, after enolization and epoxide opening, as the isomeric γ-hydroxy-α,β-enone Michael

Table 1. Intracellular replication of *T. gondii* in cultured L929 cells in-vitro.

Drug	Activity/toxicity	Dose (µM)	Inhibition at 24 h (% of control)
Atovaquone	activity	0·1	78·4
		1·0	95·2
		16·0	95·7
	toxicity	0·1	15·6
		1·0	17·4
		10·0	18·3
Artemisinin	activity	0·1	29·6
		1·0	75·8
		10·0	75·8
	toxicity	0·1	8·6
		1·0	10·3
		10·0	7·7
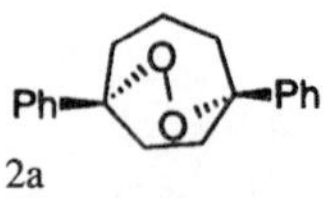 2a	activity	0·1	30·8
		1·0	69·6
		10·0	77·6
	toxicity	0·1	0·3
		1·0	0·0
		10·0	0·0
		50·0	31·2

Data from NIH, Alexandra Fairfield.

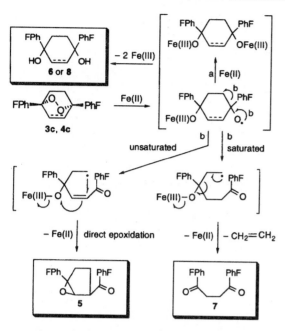

FIG. 6. Mechanism of reduction of fluorinated endoperoxides.

acceptor may kill the parasite. Likewise, saturated fluorophenyl endoperoxide **4c** may be a prodrug, activated by iron(II) to release ethylene that could be oxidized by the malaria parasite's cytochrome oxidase enzymes into ethylene oxide, an extremely reactive and damaging alkylating agent (Ortiz de Montellano 1985).

Saturated bicyclic [2·2·2] endoperoxide **4c** has very recently been found to have measurable activity in an in-vivo rodent malaria model (Peters et al 1993). Thus, this fluorinated endoperoxide **4c**, as well as bicyclic [3·2·2] endoperoxide **2a**, is a prototype suggesting strongly that fine-tuning of chemical structure to maximize the in-vivo antiparasitic therapeutic index is a worthy goal of great practical potential. We are actively pursuing this goal. Small samples of these endoperoxides are available upon request for further biological screening.

Acknowledgements
The NIH (AI-34885) is gratefully thanked for financial support, and my many colleagues and co-workers (whose names appear in the references) are thanked for their intellectual contributions and their laboratory skills. We thank Professor Peters and Dr Robinson for in-vivo testing of endoperoxide **4c**.

References

Avery, M. A., Fan, P., Karle, J. M., Bank, J. D., Miller, R., Goins, D. K. (1996) Structure-activity relationships of the antimalarial agent artemisinin. 3. Total synthesis of (+)-13-carbaartemisinin and related tetra- and tricyclic structures. J. Med. Chem. 39: 1885

Cumming, J. N., Ploypradith, P., Posner, G. H. (1996) Antimalarial activity of artemsinin (qinghaosu) and related trioxanes: mechanism(s) of action. Adv. Pharmacol. 37: 253–296

Fishwick, J., McLean, W. G., Edwards, G., Ward, S. A. (1995) The toxicity of artemisinin and related compounds on neuronal and glial cells in culture. Chem. Biol. Interact. 96: 263–271

Goldsmith, R. S. (1992) Antiprotozoal drugs, In: Katzung, B. G. (ed.) Basic and Clinical Pharmacology. Appleton & Lange, Norwalk, CT, p. 735

Meshnick, S. R., Taylor, T. E., Kamchonwongpaisan, S. (1996) Artemisinin and the antimalarial endoperoxides: from herbal remedy to targeted chemotherapy. Microbiol. Rev. 60: 301–315

Ortiz de Montellano, P. R. (1985) Chapter 5. In: Anders, M. W. (ed.) Bioactivation of Foreign Compounds. Academic Press, New York, p. 121–155

Ou-Yang, K., Krug, E. C., Marr, J. J., Berens, R. L. (1990) Inhibition of growth of *Toxoplasma gondii* by qinghaosu and derivatives. Antimicrob. Agents Chemother. 34: 1961–1965

Peters, W., Robinson, B. L., Tovey, G., Rossier, J. C., Jefford, C. W. (1993) The chemotherapy of rodent malaria. L. The activities of some synthetic 1,2,4-trioxanes against chloroquine-sensitive and chloroquine-resistant parasites. Part 3: observations on 'fenozan-50F', a difluorinated 3,3'-spirocyclopentane 1,2,4-trioxane. Ann. Trop. Med. Parasitol. 87: 111–123

Posner, G. H., Oh, C. H., Wang, D., Gerena, L., Milhous, W. K., Meshnick, S. R., Asawamahasakda, W. (1994) Mechanism-based design, synthesis, and in vitro antimalarial testing of new 4-methylated trioxanes structurally related to artemisinin: the importance of a carbon-centered radical for antimalarial activity. J. Med. Chem. 37: 1256–1258

Posner, G. H., Cumming, J. N., Ploypradith, P., Oh, C. H. (1995) Evidence for Fe(IV)=O in the molecular mechanism of action of the trioxane antimalarial artemisinin. J. Am. Chem. Soc. 117: 5885–5886

Posner, G. H., Wang, D. W., Gonzlez, L., Tao, X., Cumming, J. N., Klinedinst, D., Shapiro, T. A. (1996a) Mechanism-based design of simple, symmetrical, easily prepared, potent antimalarial endoperoxides. Tetrahedron Lett. 37: 815–818

Posner, G. H., Tao, X., Cumming, J. N., Klinedinst, D., Shapiro, T. A. (1996b) Antimalarially potent, easily prepared, fluorinated endoperoxides. Tetrahedron Lett. 37: 7225–7228

Sweeney, T. R. (1981) The present status of malaria chemotherapy: mefloquine, a novel antimalarial. Med. Res. Rev. 1: 281–301

Zhou, W. S., Xu, X. X. (1994) Total synthesis of the antimalarial sesquiterpene peroxide qinghaosu and yingzhaosu A. Acc. Chem. Res. 27: 211–216

J. Pharm. Pharmacol. 1997, 49 (Suppl. 2): 59–64

The Treatment of Malaria with Iron Chelators

ROBERT C. HIDER AND ZUDONG LIU

Department of Pharmacy, King's College London, Campden Hill Road, London W8 7AH, UK

New routes to chemotherapeutic attack on malaria are urgently required as drug resistant mutants to the antifolate pyrimethamine and the quinine family are becoming widespread. Without new drugs, falciparum malaria could become an untreatable disease in some regions within the next decade.

The idea that iron chelation might have antiplasmodial effect emerged from the awareness that many microbial pathogens depend on host-derived iron for virulence. In 1982 it was demonstrated by Pollack and co-workers that desferrioxamine possessed an antiplasmodial effect in-vitro (Raventos-Suarez et al 1982). Some years later this was followed by a clinical trial of iron-chelation therapy in children with cerebral malaria (Gordeuk et al 1992a). Desferrioxamine quickly reduced the symptoms of parasitaemia. Thus it is possible that iron chelation offers a novel approach to controlling malaria infections.

The Biology of the Erythrocyte-bound Stage

The schizont exists in the erythrocyte and it is this stage which is severely influenced by iron chelation. Merozoites released from the hepatic schizonts or from asexual blood-stage schizonts interact with uninfected red cells (erythrocytes). The invasion is highly specific, the parasite producing a parasitophorous vacuole membrane (PVM) which is continuous with the red cell membrane. Once surrounded by the PVM the parasite becomes encapsulated within the red cells cytosol (Fig. 1) (Pasvol et al 1992).

The membrane of the parasitized red cell differs in many respects from that of the parent membrane and presumably the new parasite proteins and lipids are introduced via the PVM while it remains fused to the original red cell membrane. The parasite (schizont) possesses a high metabolic activity, in contrast to the host erythrocyte and therefore nutrients need to

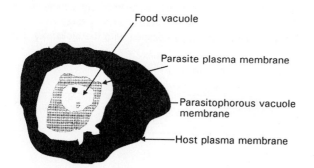

FIG. 1. Malaria parasite in the trophozoite stage. Pharmaceuticals have to permeate three membranes to gain access to the cytoplasm of the parasite.

Correspondence: R. C. Hider, Department of Pharmacy, King's College London, Campden Hill Road, London W8 7AH, UK.

be acquired and waste products removed. The rate of glycolysis can be up to 50 times that of the uninfected erythrocyte. The growing parasite degrades glucose, almost quantitatively, to lactate and, as the tricarboxylic acid cycle is absent, lactate is not oxidized further and has to be excreted. Several transport channels and proteins are located in the erythrocyte membrane which are not present in the uninfected cell (Cabantchik 1989; Elford et al 1996). The function of these proteins is to facilitate the uptake of nutrients and efflux of waste materials, a classic example being that of lactate efflux. These facilitative transport systems offer routes for selectively targeting chemotherapeutic agents including iron chelators.

The parasite, once engulfed in the erythrocyte, develops into the trophozoite stage, and uses host haemoglobin as a major nutrient source. Access to haemoglobin is achieved via the bridging structure, the cytosome. Haemoglobin-containing vesicles are pinched off from the cytostome and fuse with digestive vacuoles. Degradation occurs in these vacuoles at the pH range 5·0–5·5, the process being initiated by an aspartic proteases which clip the intact haemoglobin molecule. The resulting polypeptides are then hydrolysed to their constituent amino acids by parasite-specific hydrolysis (Goldberg et al 1990). During this process haem is released and accumulates as crystalline particles (haemozoin). Haemozoin is a polymer of haem groups linked between the central ferric iron of one haem and the carboxylate side group of another. The parasite thereby avoids the toxicity normally associated with soluble haem groups. Between 25 and 75% of the haemoglobin in an erythrocyte is degraded in this manner. Thus, with a serious malaria infection (20% parasitaemia), up to 100 g of haemoglobin is used during each cycle. These events continue for about 36 h leading to pigmented trophozoites which almost fill the erythrocyte. A phase of multiplication (schizogony), follows when the nucleus of the parasite undergoes repeated divisions, portions of the cytoplasm aggregating around the daughter nuclei to form up to 24 merozoites. After a further 48 h the envelope of the exhausted erythrocyte bursts and the merozoites are liberated into the plasma, where they attack fresh erythrocytes and the cycle is repeated.

Iron is essential for parasitic growth and multiplication, a particularly critical enzyme being ribonucleotide reductase, which is an iron-containing metalloenzyme essential for DNA synthesis (Stubbe 1990). Thus if iron-specific chelators can be selectively directed to infected erythrocytes, then a new form of chemotherapy becomes possible.

Iron Chelators as Antimalarials

Adrien Albert was the first to realize the potential of iron chelators as chemotherapeutic agents and over the period 1945–1955 he produced much data indicating the potential of bidentate ligands such as 8-hydroxyquinoline (**1**), 1-hydroxy-

Table 1.   Inhibition of *P. falciparum* by iron chelators.

Compound	ED50 (M)
8-Hydroxyquinoline (**1**)	$8\cdot3 \times 10^{-9}$
2-Methyl-8-hydroxyquinoline	$1\cdot2 \times 10^{-6}$
5-Methyl-8-hydroxyquinoline	$3\cdot1 \times 10^{-8}$
1-Hydroxypyridin-2-thione (**3**)	$7\cdot9 \times 10^{-10}$
1-Hydroxyquinolin-2-thione (**8**)	$1\cdot3 \times 10^{-7}$

ED50 is the concentration required to reduce in-vitro growth of *P. falciparum* by 50% after exposure for 3 days (Scheibel & Adler 1980, 1982)

pyridin-2-one (**2**) and 1-hydroxypyridin-2-thione (**3**) (Albert et al 1956) (Table 1). Albert pointed out that potent antibacterial molecules required a high stability constant for iron (III) and a high partition coefficient to facilitate cell penetration; he postulated that the 1:1 iron/ligand complex was toxic. This concept was applied to *P. falciparum* by Scheibel and Adler in the early 1980s (Scheibel & Adler 1982) when they considered a range of 8-hydroxyquinoline and 1-hydroxypyridin-2-thione analogues, together with diethyldithiocarbamate. As a result of these studies, compounds with similar in-vitro potency to that of quinine were identified, for instance 1 hydroxyquinolin-2-thione (**4**). A summary of these early results is presented in Table 1. Significantly the smallest compounds (**1**) and (**3**) are the most potent, a finding which contrasts with the bacteriostatic properties of the same series, where lipophilicity is critically important, the more lipophilic ligands being the most toxic (Scheibel & Adler 1982). Significantly there is a much

larger drop in inhibitory properties of 8-hydroxyquinoline when a methyl function is introduced close to the chelating centre, namely 2-methyl in contrast, to 5-methyl, the latter inducing only a slight reduction (Scheibel & Adler 1980). These results are best interpreted as the ligands exerting their activity by inhibiting a critically important metalloenzyme.

Following this work, it soon became apparent that hydrophilic iron chelators also possess antimalarial activity under both in-vivo and in-vitro conditions, this series of studies being pioneered by Raventos-Suarez et al (1982). Desferrioxamine (**5**) was found to possess an ED50 value of 10 μM and yet possesses a low K_{part} value. Furthermore desferrioxamine was found to induce a powerful stage-dependent inhibitory effect. Table 2 shows hypoxanthine incorporation, as a measure of growth by parasites. Exposure to desferrioxamine in 8 h pulses during the first 23 h, when the parasites were between ring and non-pigmented trophozoite stages had no inhibitory effect on growth. In contrast exposure to desferrioxamine after 23 h, when the parasites had matured into pigmented trophozoites and schizonts, resulted in more than 50% supression of hypoxanthine incorporation (Whitehead & Peto 1990). Thus sensitivity to iron chelation occurs late in the parasite cycle and coincides with the period of maximum DNA synthesis. This renders ribonucleotide reductase as a likely target for inhibition by hydrophilic iron chelators. A wider variety of iron chelators are known to inhibit ribonucleotide reductase (Ganeshaguru et al 1980; Cory et al 1981).

Subsequent to these key investigations, a diverse range of iron chelators has been demonstrated to possess antimalarial activity. These include: *tris*-hydroxamate siderophores including tripodal hydroxamates (**6**) (Shanzer et al 1991; Lytton et al 1993); 3-hydroxy-pyridin-4-ones (**7**) (Heppner et al 1988; Hershko et al 1992); phenolic and catecholic ligands including HBED (**8**) (Yinnan et al 1989); pyridoxal betaines (Tsafack et al 1996); desferrithiocin (**9**) (Fritsch et al 1987); and daphnetin, a dihydroxycoumarin (**10**) (Yang et al 1992).

Significantly, extracts from the bark of ash trees, which are rich in coumarins have been used as folk remedies to treat malaria in China (Steck 1971). Daphnetin is currently being used clinically in China to treat Bruger's disease, a coagulation disorder (Li 1986).

Mode of Action of Antimalarial Iron Chelators

There is no clear consensus of the mode of action of iron chelators and this is almost certainly because there are several potential toxic pathways associated with the molecules. It is

Table 2.   [³H]Hypoxanthine uptake by *P. falciparum* following exposure to desferrioxamine.

Exposure time (h)	Hypoxanthine uptake at 42 h (% control)
0–7	100
7–15	84
15–23	102
23–30	51
30 +	37
0–42	28

The concentration of desferrioxamine was 100 μM. N = 6 (Peto & Thompson 1986).

likely that chelators with different physical and chemical properties possess different modes of action, relevant properties being: hydrophobicity; size and stereochemistry in the immediate vicinity of the chelating function; redox stability of ligand; and redox stability of iron complex.

Deprivation of parasite iron source

The precise iron source for the malaria parasite is unknown but it has been clearly demonstrated not to be of extracellular origin for *P. falciparum* (Peto & Thompson 1986). The growth rate of the parasite is not influenced by the iron status of the host. When parasites invade erythrocytes they generate a low molecular weight iron pool (Hershko & Peto 1988) which must originate from haemoglobin digestion. Exposure to powerful iron chelators would limit the size of this pool, thereby reducing the rate of incorporation of iron into critical redox proteins and metalloenzymes. This mechanism is likely to be associated with the larger water soluble hexadentate chelators, for instance desferrioxamine (5), synthetic trihydroxamates (6) and HBED (8). Some of the more water soluble bidentate ligands, for instance the 3-hydroxypyridin-4-ones (7) may also operate via this mechanism. Control of membrane permeation is a key factor in the efficacy of such molecules and this has been systematically investigated by Lytton et al (1993) with hexadentate ligands and Hershko et al (1992) with bidentate ligands. Both groups found a close relationship between the ability to penetrate the infected erythrocyte membrane by simple diffusion and efficacy of the antimalarial effect. The assignment of this mode of action to desferrioxamine is consistent with its proven ability to inhibit ribonucleotide reductase, there being an appreciable time lag between the entry of the cell by desferrioxamine and inhibition of the enzyme (Cooper et al 1996).

Activation of haemozoin-iron

The stable crystalline structure of haemozoin is critically important for the viability of the parasite, the dissociated haem being potentially toxic due to the generation of hydroxyl radicals under aerobic conditions. Van Zyl et al (1993) proposed that desferrioxamine somehow disrupts the haemozoin complex, thereby generating toxic levels of the dissociated haem moieties. More direct evidence is required for this interesting proposal. Significantly the highly effective peroxide-containing antimalarial artemisinin is also reported to be dependent on haemozoin (Meshnick et al 1993). The polymeric haem is believed to activate artemisinin yielding toxic radicals. It should be noted however that both desferrioxamine (5) and 3-hydroxypyridinones (7) inhibit the antimalarial activity of artemisinin (Meshnick et al 1993). It is conceivable therefore that the selectivity of artemisinin for infected erythrocytes is not associated with the presence of haemozoin, but rather the elevated level of low molecular weight iron complexes.

Direct generation of hydroxyl radicals due to the presence of a toxic iron complex

This mechanism dates back to Albert (Albert et al 1956) and undoubtedly will occur with the hydrophobic bidentate ligands such as the substituted 8-hydroxyquinolines and possibly extremely hydrophobic 3-hydroxypyridin-4-ones (7). Unfortunately it is unlikely that this mode of action will be parasite-

selective, highly potent molecules also being toxic to the host. In contrast, hexadentate compounds such as desferrioxamine (5), HBED (8) and the synthetic tris-hydroxamates (6) will not generate hydroxyl radicals in the presence of iron (III) as they form extremely stable non toxic complexes.

Direct inhibition of metalloenzymes

There are a number of important iron-containing enzymes which are potential targets for iron chelation. In general chelating agents are unable to form stable ternary complexes or remove the iron from haem-containing and iron-sulphur enzymes. In contrast enzymes with iron co-ordinated to oxygen ligands appear to be more susceptible, for instance ribonucleotide reductase and lipoxygenase. As the malaria parasite is a rapidly proliferating organism, particularly at the late trophozoite stage, optimal activity of ribonucleotide reductase is essential for DNA synthesis.

The iron centre of this enzyme is co-ordinated directly to the polypeptide backbone and is located approximately 5Å distant from the essential tyrosine radical. The crystal structure of the *Escherichia coli* enzyme demonstrates that the iron centre is not readily assessable to the surrounding aqueous phase (Nordlund et al 1990). Consequently, it is likely that only small, non bulky ligands can gain access to the iron centre. 3-Hydroxypyridin-4-ones (7) and 8-hydroxyquinoline (1) together with the 1-hydroxypyridin-2-ones (2) and -thiones (3) are likely candidates.

The influence of 3-hydroxypyridin-4-ones on the cell cycle has been intensively studied by Porter and co-workers (Hoyes et al 1992). By inhibiting ribonucleotide reductase these ligands reversibly inhibit proliferating cells in the S-phase. Removal of the chelator after brief exposure leads to the complete recovery of cells. In addition to this indirect evidence for inhibition of ribonucleotide reductase, ESR measurements of the tyrosine radical signal confirms such inhibition. Indeed, in contrast to desferrioxamine, 3-hydroxypyridin-4-ones inhibit this enzyme extremely rapidly (Cooper et al 1996), which is indicative of a direct inhibition, either by ternary complex formation, removal of the essential iron at the active site of the enzyme, or by quenching the tyrosine radical. The former is more likely, in so far as the inhibitory effect induced by the pyridinones can be rapidly reversed (Hoyes et al 1992).

Use of Desferrioxamine in Man

Desferrioxamine is the only pharmaceutical which is available for the treatment of iron-overload (Porter 1989). As a result, it is widely prescribed for transfusion-dependent thalassaemic patients. Due to its poor ability to penetrate mammalian cells, it is relatively non toxic. However, in contrast to normal erythrocytes, desferrioxamine is capable of entering parasitized cells (Scott et al 1990) and therefore does have potential for limiting parasite proliferation.

As a result of the finding that desferrioxamine given by constant subcutaneous infusion suppresses parasitaemia in *P. falciparum*-infected *Aotus* monkeys (Pollack et al 1987), Gordeuk and co-workers undertook a small clinical trial in Zambia (Gordeuk et al 1992b). Desferrioxamine was administered at a rate of 100 mg kg^{-1}/24 h by continous 72 h subcutaneous infusion to 28 volunteers with asymptomatic *P. falciparum* infection in a randomized, double-blind, placebo-controlled cross-over trial. A significant decrease in concentration of asexual intraerythrocyte parasites was induced by desferrioxamine. However parasitaemia recurred in the majority of the volunteers over the following 6 months. A parallel study was undertaken in Thailand using an identical dose (Bunnag et al 1992), but with half the patients suffering from symptomatic *P. vivax* infection and the other half from uncomplicated *P. falciparum* infection. In both groups desferrioxamine reduced the parasitaemia to zero within 106 and 57 h and with fever clearance times of 55–60 h, respectively. Again parasitaemia recurred in the majority of patients.

The results of these two studies are summarized in Table 3. Clearly the intravenous route is more effective than the subcutaneous route. The likely explanation is the achievement of higher serum concentrations with intravenous than with subcutaneous administration, the respective concentrations being 7 and 20 μM. The latter value is close to the ID50 value for desferrioxamine against *P. falciparum* determined in-vitro (Mabeza et al 1996). The influence of desferrioxamine on cerebral malaria has also been investigated by Gordeuk and co-workers (1992a). Unrousable coma in severe *P. falciparum* infections is associated with mortality of about 15% in children and 20% in adults (much higher mortality rates are recorded in Africa). In fatal cases the cerebral capillaries and venules are packed with erythrocytes containing malaria parasites, which adhere to the vascular endothelium. The brain becomes ischaemic. A double-blind placebo-controlled study of desferrioxamine (100 mg kg^{-1} (24 h)$^{-1}$, i.v.) in 83 Zambian children suffering from severe falciparum malaria and all being treated with a standard quinine-based regime was undertaken (Gordeuk et al 1992a). Recovery of full consciousness was more rapid with desferrioxamine and the rate of clearance of parasites was also enhanced in the presence of the chelator. Among 50 children with deep coma, the estimated median recovery times were 68 h with placebo and 24 h with desferrioxamine. In addition to the possibility that desferrioxamine possesses a direct antiplasmodial action, the chelator could have a protective effect on cerebral tissue. Hydroxyl radical damage occurs under ischaemic conditions and iron-induced radicals enhance this damage. Iron chelation with desferrioxamine might therefore be expected to reduce such activity (Mabeza et al 1996).

Table 3. The influence of desferrioxamine (100mgkg^{-1}) on parasitaemia in patients infected with two different Plasmodium.

	Time to reduce parasitaemia (h)			n of study	Country
	50%	90%	100%		
P. falciparum					
Desferrioxamine (s.c.)	28	39	104	16	Zambia
Desferrioxamine (i.v.)	9	25	48	14	Thailand
P. vivax					
Desferrioxamine (i.v.)	17	39	72	14	Thailand

Mabeza et al (1996).

It is clear from the studies that iron chelators have the capacity to clear parasites under clinical conditions. Unfortunately desferrioxamine is not orally active (Hider et al 1994).

Recrudescence
As indicated by the clinical studies with desferrioxamine there is apparently quite extensive recrudenscence. This probably results from the chelator blocking cell cycling of the parasite but not causing death. This particular aspect of iron chelator activity has been studied in detail by Cabantchik and co-workers (Golenser et al 1995; Cabantchik et al 1996). Irreversible damage can be induced in the malaria parasite by the simultaneous use of two chelators, typically one being hydrophilic and the other hydrophobic and therefore highly permeable to the parasite. It is argued that by adversely influencing iron supply to all the three stages, parasite death occurs (Golenser et al 1995) and therefore recrudence will be absent. A successful synergy was observed in-vitro for desferrioxamine and certain tripodal tris hydroxamates (Golenser et al 1995).

Possible Design for Orally Active Iron Chelators

There are several critical features of an iron chelator which endow it with good oral absorption, and these have been recently reviewed (Hider et al 1994). Basically, the molecular weight should be less than 250 and ideally the ligand should be neutral. Thus bidentate ligands of the type (**1, 2, 3** and **7**) are ideal for oral absorption. Of these, the 3-hydroxypyridin-4-ones have been most extensively investigated (Porter et al

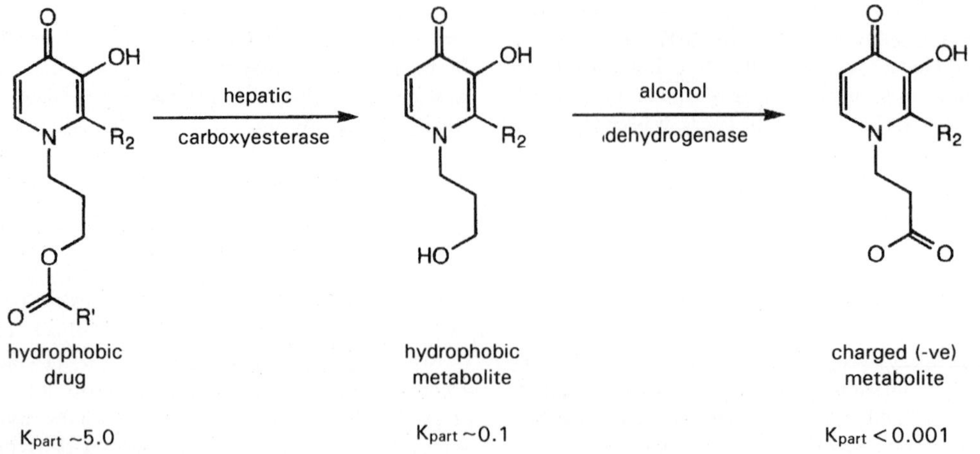

Scheme 1. Prodrug approach to antimalarial agents.

1990; Dobbin et al 1993). Unfortunately many of the molecules with good antimalarial activity are also toxic to mammalian cells (Hershko et al 1992). The one exception so far tested is CP38 (7, $R_1 = CH_2CH_2CO_2H$, $R_2 = CH_3$) which is an inhibitor of *P. falciparum* but relatively non-toxic to mammalian cells. The partition coefficient (water/n-octanol) for CP38 is extremely low endowing the molecule with poor ability to penetrate membranes (Porter et al 1988) and therefore it is likely that CP38 enters parasitized erythrocytes via a carrier-mediated mechanism, possibly the lactate carrier (Kanaani & Ginsburg 1991, 1992). Thus it may prove possible to specifically target 3-hydroxypyridin-4-ones to the malaria parasite.

In support of the proposal that the anionic CP38 penetrates the infected erythrocyte by facilitated diffusion, is the finding that the property is limited to a well defined structure. Thus in a study of the ability to inhibit the growth of *P. falciparum* by a range of anionic hydroxypyridinones, only CP38 and CP110 possessed ED50 values in the range of 50 μM (Table 4).

Table 4. Structure and ED50 values of 3-hydroxypyridin-4-ones (7) for the in-vitro inhibition of *P. falciparum*.

Hydroxypyridinone	R_1	R_2	ED50 (μM)
CP20	CH_3	CH_3	67
CP38	$CH_2CH_2CO_2H$	CH_3	56
CP110	$CH_2CH_2CO_2H$	$CH_2 CH_3$	53
CP31	CH_2CO_2H	CH_3	370
CP39	$CH_2CH_2CH_2CO_2H$	CH_3	250
CP85	$CH_2CH_2SO_3H$	CH_3	650

Although this value is much higher than those corresponding to conventional antimalarials, the anionic iron chelators (CP38 and CP110) are much less toxic to mammalian cells and levels of 50 μM are clinically attainable with oral administration of related hydroxypyridone CP20 (Kontoghiorghes et al 1990). Unfortunately, although CP20 possesses some antimalarial properties under in-vitro conditions, it lacks such activity when used clinically (Mabeza et al 1996) due to its extremely rapid metabolism (Singh et al 1992). CP38 and CP110, unlike CP20, are not glucuronidated by mammalian tissue.

Not surprisingly the very property that renders CP38 non-toxic to mammalian cells, leads to relatively poor oral absorption. In principle, this difficulty can be circumvented by the prodrug concept, utilising the ability of the liver to efficiently metabolize pyridinones (Hider et al 1996). A typical sequence of reactions which occurs in high yield in both rodents and man is depicted in Scheme 1. The prodrug ester is absorbed from the intestine with high efficiency. Molecules of this class are currently being investigated for their ability to function as antimalarials in in-vivo models.

References

Albert, A., Rees, C. W., Tomlinson, A. J. H. (1956) Why are metal binding substances anti-bacterial? Recueil 75: 819–824

Bunnag, D., Poltera, A. A., Viravan, C., Looareesuwan, S., Harinasuta, K. T., Schindlery, C. (1992) Plasmodicidal effect of desferrioxamine-β in human vivax or falciparum malaria from Thailand. Acta Trop. 52: 59–67

Cabantchik, Z. I. (1989) Altered membrane transport of malaria-infected erythrocytes: a possible pharmacological target. Blood 74: 1464–1471

Cabantchik, Z. I., Glickstein, H., Golenser, J., Loyevsky, M., Tsafack, A. (1996) Iron chelators: mode of action as antimalarials. Acta Haematol. 95: 70–77

Cooper, C. E., Lynagh, G. R., Hoyes, K. P., Hider, R. C., Cammack, R., Porter, J. B. (1996) The relationship of intracellular iron chelation to the inhibition and regeneration of human ribonucleotide reductase. J. Biol. Chem. 271: 20291–20299

Cory, J. G., Lasater, L., Sato, A. (1981) Effect of iron chelating agents on inhibitors of ribonucleotide reductase. Biochem. Pharmacol. 30: 979–984

Dobbin, P. S., Hider, R. C., Hall, A. D., Taylor, P. D., Sarpong, P., Porter, J. B., Xiao, G., Van Der Helm, D. (1993) Synthesis, physicochemical properties and biological evaluation of N-substituted 2-alkyl-3-hydroxy-4(1H)pyridinones: orally active iron chelators with clinical potential. J. Med. Chem. 36: 2448–2548

Elford, B. C., Cowan, G. M., Ferguson, J. P. (1996) Parasite-regulated membrane transport processes and metabolic control in malaria-infected erythrocytes. Biochem. J. 308: 361–374

Fritsch, G., Sawatzki, G., Treumer, J., Jung, A., Spira, D. R. (1987) *Plasmodium falciparum*: inhibition in vitro with lactoferrin, desferrithiocin and desferricrocin. Exp. Parasitol. 63: 1

Ganeshaguru, K., Hoffbrand, A. V., Grady, R. W., Cerami, A. (1980) Effect of iron chelating agents on DNA synthesis in human cells. Biochem. Pharmacol. 29: 1275–1279

Goldberg, D. E., Slater, A. F. G., Cerami, A., Henderson, G. B. (1990) Haemoglobin degradation in the malaria parasite *Plasmodium falciparum*: an ordered process in a unique organelle. Proc. Natl Acad. Sci. USA 87: 2931–2935

Golenser, J., Tsafack, A., Amichai, Y., Libman, J., Shanzer, A., Cabantchik, Z. I. (1995) Antimalarial action of hydroxamate-based iron chelators and potentiation of desferrioxamine action by reversed siderophores. Antimicrob. Agents Chemother. 39: 61–65

Gordeuk, V., Thuma, P., Brittenham, G., McLaren, C., Parry, D., Backenstrose, A., Biemba, G., Msiska, R., Holmes, L., McKinlye, E., Vargas, L., Gilkeson, R., Poltera, A. A. (1992a) Effect of iron chelation therapy of recovery from deep coma in children with cerebral malaria. N. Engl. J. Med. 237: 1473–1477

Gordeuk, Y. R., Thuma, P. E., Brittenham, G. M., Zulu, S., Simwanza, G., Mhang, A., Flesch, G., Parry, D. (1992b) Iron chelation with desferrioxamine β in adults with asymptomatic *Plasmodium falciparum* parasitemia. Blood 79: 308–312

Heppner, D. G., Hallaway, P. E., Kontoghiorghes, G. J., Eaton, J. W. (1988) Antimalarial properties of orally active iron chelators. Blood 72: 358–361

Hershko, C., Peto, T. E. A. (1988) Desferrioxamine inhibition of malaria is independent of host iron status. J. Exp. Med. 168: 375

Hershko, C., Gordeuk, V. R., Thuma, P. E., Theanacho, E. N., Spira, D. T., Hider, R. C., Peto, T. E. A., Brittenham, G. M. (1992) The antimalarial effect of iron chelator studies in animal models and in humans with mild falciparum malaria. J. Inorg. Biochem. 47: 267–277

Hider, R. C., Porter, J. B., Singh, S. (1994) The design of therapeutically useful iron chelators. In: Bergeron, R. J., Brittenham, G. M. (eds) The Design of Therapeutically Useful Iron Chelators in the Development of Iron Chelators for Clinical Use. CRC Press, Ann Arbor, pp 353–371

Hider, R. C., Choudhury, R., Rai, B. I., Dehkordi, L. S., Singh, S. (1996) Design of orally active iron chelators. Eur. J. Drug Metab. Disposit. 95: 6–12

Hoyes, K. P., Hider, R. C., Porter, J. B. (1992) Cell cycle synchronisation and growth inhibition by 3-hydroxypyridin-4-one iron chelators in leukamia cell lines. Cancer Res. 52: 4591–4599

Kannani, J., Ginsburg, H. (1991) Transport of lactate in *Plasmodium falciparum*-infected human erythrocytes. J. Cell Physiol. 149: 469–476

Kannani, J., Ginsburg, H. (1992) Effect of cinnamic acid derivatives on *in vitro* growth of *Plasmodium falciparum* and on the permeability of the membrane of malaria-infected erythrocytes. Antimicrob. Agents Chemother. 36: 1102–1108

Kontoghiorghes, G. J., Goddard, J. G., Bartlet, A. N., Sheppard, L. (1990) Pharmacokinetic studies in humans with the oral iron chelator 1,2-dimethyl-3-hydroxypyrid-4-one. Clin. Pharmacol. Ther. 48: 255–261

Li, X.-M. (1986) Clinical analysis of the efficacy of daphnetin in the treatment of Bruger's disease in 112 cases. Jilin Med. 7: 28–29

Lytton, S. D., Mester, B., Dayan, I., Glickstein, H., Libman, J., Shanzer, A., Cabantchik, Z. I. (1993) Mode of action of iron(III) chelators as antimalarials: 1. Membrane permeation properties and cytotoxic activity. Blood 81: 214–221

Mabeza, G. F., Biemba, G., Gordeuk, V. R. (1996) Clinical studies of iron chelators in malaria. Acta Haematol. 95: 78–86

Meshnik, S. R., Yang, Y. Z., Lima, V., Kuypers, F., Kamchonwongpaisan, S., Yuthovong, Y. (1993) Iron-dependent free radical generation from the antimalarial agent artemisinin (Quinghasosu). Antimicrob. Agents Chemother. 37: 1108–1114

Nordlund, P., Sjoberg, B. M., Eklund, H. (1990) Three-dimensional structure of the free radical protein of ribonucleotide reductase. Nature 345: 593–598

Pasvol, G., Cough, B., Carlsson, J. (1992) Malaria and the red cell membrane. Blood Reviews 6: 183–192

Pattanapanyasat, K., Thaithong, S., Kyle, D. E., Udomsangpetch, R., Yongvanitchit, K., Hider, R. C., Webster, H. K. (1997) Flow cytometric assessment of hydroxypyridinone iron chelators on in vitro growth of drug-resistant malaria. Cytometry In press

Peto, T. E. A., Thompson, J. L. (1986) A reappraisal of the effects iron and desferrioxamine on the growth of Plasmodium falciparum in vitro: the unimportance of serum iron. Br. J. Haematol. 63: 273–280

Pollack, S., Rossan, R. N., Davidson, D. E., Escajadillo, A. (1987) Desferrioxamine suppresses Plasmodium falciparum in Aotus monkeys. Proc. Soc. Exp. Biol. Med. 184: 162–164

Porter, J. B. (1989) Oral iron chelators; prospects for future development. Eur. J. Haematol. 43: 271–285

Porter, J. B., Gyparaki, M., Burke, L. C., Huehns, E. R., Sarpong, P., Saez, V., Hider, R. C. (1988) Iron mobilization from hepatocyte monolayer cultures by chelators: the importance of membrane permeability and the iron-binding constant. Blood 72: 1497–1503

Porter, J. B., Morgan, J., Hoyes, K. P., Burke, L. C., Huehns, E. R., Hider, R. C. (1990) Relative efficacy and acute toxicity of hydroxypyridin-4-one iron chelators in mice. Blood 76: 2389–2396

Raventos-Suarez, C., Pollack, S., Nagal, R. L. (1982) Plasmodium falciparum: inhibition of in-vitro growth by deferoxamine. Am. J. Trop. Med. Hyg. 31: 919–922

Scheibel, L. W., Adler, A. (1980) Antimalarial activity of selected aromatic chelators. Mol. Pharmacol. 18: 320–325

Scheibel, L. W., Adler, A. (1982) III 8-Hydroxyquinolines (oxines) substituted in position 5 and 7 and oxines annelated in position 5, 6 by an aromatic ring. Mol. Pharmacol. 22: 140–144

Scott, M. D., Ranz, A., Kuypers, F. A., Lubin, B. H., Meshnick, S. R. (1990) Parasite uptake of desferrioxamine: a prerequisite for antimalarial activity. Br. J. Haematol. 75: 598–602

Shanzer, A., Libman, J., Lytton, S. D., Glickstein, H., Cabantchik, Z. I. (1991) Reversed siderophores act as antimalarial agents. Proc. Natl Acad. Sci. USA 88: 6585–6589

Singh, S., Epemolu, R. O., Dobbin, P. S., Tilbrook, G. S., Ellis, B. L., Damani, L. A., Hider, R. C. (1992) Urinary metabolic profiles in human and rat of 1,2-dimethyl- and 1,2-diethyl-substituted 3-hydroxypyridin-4-ones. Drug Metab. Dispos. 20: 256–261

Steck, E. (1971) The Chemotherapy of Protozoal Diseases. Walter Reed Army Institute of Research, Washington DC

Stubbe, J. (1990). Ribonucleotide reductases: amazing and confusing. J. Biol. Chem. 265: 5329–5332

Tsafack, A., Loyevsky, M., Ponka, P., Cabantchik, Z. I. (1996) Mode of action of iron (III) chelators as antimalarials. J. Lab. Clin. Med. 127: 574–582

Van Zyl, R. L., Havlik, I., Hemplemann, E., MacPhail, A. P., McNamaro, L. (1993) Malaria pigment and excellular iron. Possible target from iron chelating agents. Biochem. Pharmacol. 45: 1431–1436

Whitehead, S., Peto, T. E. A. (1990) Stage-dependent effect of desferrioxamine on growth of Plasmodium falciparum in vitro. Blood 76: 1250–1255

Yang, Y. Z., Ranz, A., Pan, H. Z., Zhang, Z. N., Lin, X. B., Meshnick, S. R. (1992) Daphnetin: a novel antimalarial agent with in vitro and in vivo activity. Am. J. Trop. Med. Hyg. 46: 15–20

Yinnan, A. M., Theanacho, E. N., Grady, R. W., Spira, D. T., Hershko, C. (1989) Antimalarial effect of HBED and other phenolic and catecholic iron chelators. Blood 74: 2166–2171

J. Pharm. Pharmacol. 1997, 49(Suppl. 2): 65–69

Antimalarial Agents Directed at Thymidylate Synthase

PRADIPSINH K. RATHOD

Department of Biology, The Catholic University of America, Washington, D.C., 20064 USA

After many years of decline, malaria is re-emerging as a major health threat around the world (Oaks et al 1991). New treatments against *Plasmodium falciparum* are necessary because parasites are rapidly developing resistance to existing drugs (White 1996).

Many biochemical studies on protozoan parasites accentuate enzymes and metabolic pathways that are potential targets for selective chemotherapy. However, most clinically useful drugs still arise through empirical screening of natural products or synthetic analogues of previously successful antimalarial agents. The scarcity of new antimetabolites against malarial parasites is a measure of our limited ability to exploit differences in metabolic pathways between mammalian cells and malarial parasites for selective chemotherapy.

Recently, it has been possible to identify potent and selective antimalarial agents by directing antimetabolites at malarial thymidylate synthase.

Rationale for Targeting Thymidylate Synthase

Pyrimidine metabolism in malaria

The erythrocytic phase of the life cycle of *P. falciparum* is associated with the clinical symptoms of malaria. During this 48 h cycle, each parasite inside a red blood cell generates about 24 offspring that burst out and reinvade new host cells. The exponential increase in parasite DNA and RNA requires a proportional supply of purine and pyrimidine nucleotides. Malarial parasites use the rich pool of adenine nucleotides in erythrocytes to obtain purines, but the parasites have to synthesize pyrimidines de novo (Gutteridge & Trigg 1970; Sherman 1979; Reyes et al 1982).

Erythrocytic stages of malarial parasites are completely dependent on the de novo pyrimidine pathway. Malarial parasites fail to incorporate exogenous radiolabelled pyrimidine bases and pyrimidine nucleosides into nucleic acids (Gutteridge & Trigg 1970; Sherman 1979). Additionally, erythrocytic stages of *P. falciparum* are rich in enzymes for de novo pyrimidine biosynthesis but lack the enzymes for salvage of pyrimidine bases or nucleosides (Reyes et al 1982). Orotic acid, an intermediate in de novo pyrimidine biosynthesis, can be metabolized by malarial parasites (Gutteridge & Trigg 1970; Reyes et al 1982; Rathod & Reyes 1983).

In contrast to malarial parasites, most mammalian cells have both the capacity for de novo synthesis of pyrimidine nucleosides as well as salvage of preformed pyrimidines (Jones 1980; Moyer et al 1985). On this basis, one would suspect that a potent, selective inhibitor of any of the steps in de novo pyrimidine biosynthesis would be a selective inhibitor of malarial parasite proliferation, particularly when used in combination with nucleosides. Host-parasite differences in the structure of the target enzymes would be of additional benefit but would not be entirely necessary.

Biosynthesis of thymidylate in malaria

Thymidylate synthase plays an important role in the biosynthesis of DNA precursors. Using methylenetetrahydrofolate as a co-substrate, this enzyme converts 2′-deoxyuridylate to thymidylate (Carreras & Santi 1995). Continued activity of thymidylate synthase is dependent on an active dihydrofolate reductase which regenerates tetrahydrofolate from dihydrofolate (Schweitzer et al 1990).

Dihydrofolate reductase activity and thymidylate synthase activity reside on a single polypeptide encoded by a single gene in all protozoan parasites examined (Garrett et al 1984). Malarial dihydrofolate reductase-thymidylate synthase has been cloned and sequenced (Bzig et al 1987). The bifunctional enzyme has been purified from malarial parasites in culture and from heterologous expression systems (Zolg et al 1989; Sirawaraporn et al 1990; Hekmat-Nejad & Rathod 1996).

Of all the steps in de novo pyrimidine metabolism, the biosynthesis of thymidylate appears to be a particularly attractive target for chemotherapy because, in many cell types, even partial inhibition of this step is known to result in nucleotide imbalances and cell death (Ingraham et al 1986; Yoshioka et al 1987; Houghton et al 1989; Kunz et al 1994). Selective inhibition of malarial dihydrofolate reductase by compounds such as pyrimethamine and cycloguanil is responsible for the antimalarial activity of pyrimethamine and proguanil (Carrington et al 1951; Hitchings 1960; Ferone et al 1969).

Resistance to these antimalarial agents is most frequently associated with point mutations in the dihydrofolate reductase domain of the bifunctional enzyme (Foote et al 1990; Peterson et al 1990). Pyrimethamine-resistance can be acquired via transfection of a gene encoding a pyrimethamine-resistant dihydrofolate reductase-thymidylate synthase (Donald & Roos 1993; Crabb & Cowman 1996; van Dijk et al 1996; Wu et al 1996).

Until recently, strategies for selective inhibition of malarial thymidylate synthase domain were nonexistent. The problem appeared particularly challenging because thymidylate synthase is considered to be among the most conserved protein in nature (Carreras & Santi 1995). In terms of steady-state kinetics, there are no differences between malarial and mammalian thymidylate synthase (Table 1).

5-Fluoro-2′-deoxyuridylate and thymidylate synthase

A 5-fluorinated analog of 2′-deoxyuridylate is a potent inactivator of thymidylate synthase from mammalian cells and other sources (Reyes & Heidelberger 1965; Heidelberger et al 1983; Carreras & Santi 1995). The normal mechanism of thymidylate synthase includes a tertiary complex involving covalent attachments between the enzyme thymidylate synthase, 2′-deoxyuridylate, and the co-substrate methylenetetrahydrofolate (Santi 1981). Subsequent steps in the catalytic

Table 1. A comparison of the kinetic constants of thymidylate synthase from *P. falciparum* and from mammalian cells.

Kinetic property	*P. falciparum*		Mammalian enzyme
	Recombinant enzyme	Native enzyme	
K_m, 2'-deoxyuridylate	2·0 μM	1·3 μM	1·8 μM, 3·4 μM
K_m, methylenetetrahydrofolate	39 μM	30 μM	31 μM, 8 μM, 27 μM
k_{cat}, (per FdUMP binding site)	118 min^{-1}	120 min^{-1}	150 min^{-1}
K_i, FdUMP	2·0 nM	–	1·7 nM, 5 nM
K_i, D1694 monoglutamate	2·80 μM	–	0·06 μM
K_i, D1694 pentaglutamate	1·5 nM	–	1·0 nM

Hekmat-Nejad & Rathod (1996).

reaction require extraction of a proton from the 5-position of the pyrimidine ring. In the presence of methylenetetrahydrofolate and 5-fluoro-2'-deoxyuridylate, thymidylate synthase forms an analogous ternary species but this complex is stable and fails to dissociate in the forward direction due to the fluorine in the 5-position of the pyrimidine ring.

The K_i of 5-fluoro-2'-deoxyuridylate for malarial thymidylate synthase is about 2 nM when tested in the presence of 100 μM methylenetetrahydrofolate (Table 1; Hekmat-Nejad & Rathod 1996). This value is comparable with the potency of 5-fluoro-2'-deoxyuridylate against thymidylate synthase molecules from human and other mammalian sources (Reyes & Heidelberger 1965; Dolnick & Cheng 1977; Davisson et al 1989).

Antimalarial Activity of 5-Fluoroorotate In-Vitro

Generating 5-fluoro-2'-deoxyuridylate in malarial parasites
While 5-fluoro-2'-deoxyuridylate is a potent inhibitor of thymidylate synthase, this molecule itself is not well suited for inhibiting proliferation of cells, since most cells are not permeable to nucleotides. Compounds such as 5-fluorouracil, 5-fluorouridine, and 5-fluoro-2'-deoxyuridine, which can act as metabolic precursors of 5-fluoro-2'-deoxyuridylate, are potent inhibitors of some proliferating mammalian cells. Since malarial parasites lack enzymes for salvage of standard pyrimidines such precursors were not expected to have potent antimalarial activity. Indeed, 5-fluorouracil, 5-fluorouridine, and 5-fluoro-2'-deoxyuridine are far less effective against malarial parasites than against mammalian cells in culture (Rathod et al 1989).

Based on precursor incorporation studies and enzyme profiles in *P. falciparum*, it was known that exogenous orotic acid, an intermediate in de novo pyrimidine biosynthesis, was utilized by malarial parasites. It was also known that, at least in other cells, enzymes responsible for orotic acid metabolism could convert 5-fluoroorotic acid into toxic fluorinated nucleotides. It was hypothesized that 5-fluoroorotic acid would be a potent antimalarial agent and this potency would be closely related to inactivation of malarial thymidylate synthase activity.

In-vitro activity of 5-fluoroorotate against P. falciparum
5-Fluoroorotate is a potent and selective antimalarial agent (Rathod et al 1989; Gomez & Rathod 1990). The IC50 of 5-

fluoroorotate against *P. falciparum* in culture was about 6 nM (Table 2). About 0·1 μM 5-fluoroorotate was sufficient to completely inhibit proliferation of malarial parasites in culture. Malarial parasites resistant to chloroquine, quinine, pyrimethamine, and sulphadoxine were as susceptible to 5-fluoroorotate as traditional drug-sensitive parasites (Table 2). Addition of preformed pyrimidines such as uridine to the culture medium did not alter the susceptibility of malarial parasites to 5-fluoroorotate, consistent with predictions based on precursor incorporation studies and assay of enzyme activities in malarial parasites (Reyes et al 1982).

Inactivation of malarial thymidylate synthase
Uninfected erythrocytes lack detectable thymidylate synthase, so the status of thymidylate synthase in 5-fluoroorotate treated malarial parasites could be determined by directly assaying lysates of infected erythrocytes for the ability to release tritiated water from 5-[^{3}H] deoxyuridine monophosphate (Rathod et al 1992). The same doses of 5-fluoroorotate that were sufficient to inhibit proliferation of malarial parasites were also sufficient to inactivate thymidylate synthase activity in infected erythrocytes (Rathod et al 1992). Control studies demonstrated that during the early phases of thymidylate synthase inactivation, dihydrofolate reductase on the other half of the bifunctional enzyme remained active (Rathod et al 1992). This was consistent with the hypothesis that loss of thymidylate synthase activity in 5-fluoroorotate-treated cells was specific and not due to general necrosis.

Thymidylate synthase inactivation was expected to lead to nucleotide imbalances and cell death (Ingraham et al 1986; Yoshioka et al 1987; Houghton et al 1989; Kunz et al 1994). Indeed, a clonal viability assay for *P. falciparum* was developed and it confirmed that the doses of 5-fluoroorotate that were sufficient to inhibit thymidylate synthase activity and parasite proliferation were also sufficient to kill parasites (Young & Rathod 1993). Similarly, there was a close relationship between the duration of exposure to 5-fluoroorotate necessary to inhibit thymidylate synthase and loss of cell viability.

An alternate mechanism for toxicity from 5-fluoropyrimidines involves incorporation of fluorinated nucleotides into RNA molecules (Evans et al 1980). Usually this mode of toxicity is associated with substitution of at least 2% of uridine molecules in RNA with 5-fluorouridine molecules. In malarial parasites, nanomolar concentrations of 5-fluoroorotate are not

Table 2. Antiproliferative activity of 5-fluoroorotate against *P. falciparum* and against human HT-1080 cells.

Antimalarial agent	*P. falciparum* cells		Human cells Fibrosarcoma HT-1080
	Drug-sensitive clone D6 from Sierra Leonne	Drug-resistant clone W2 from Indochina	
5-Fluoroorotate	6 nM	6 nM	10 000 nM
5-Fluoroorotate plus 1 mM uridine	6 nM	6 nM	50 000 nM

Values represent 50% inhibitory concentration. Rathod et al (1989).

sufficient to cause significant incorporation of 5-fluorouridine into parasite RNA or DNA (Rathod et al 1992).

Toxicity to mammalian cells
While the in-vitro potency of 5-fluoroorotate was encouraging, it was equally important to evaluate the potential toxicity of 5-fluoroorotate against mammalian cells in culture (Rathod et al 1989). It required higher than 1 μM 5-fluoroorotate before significant toxicity was observed against 5 different types of mammalian cells in culture. 5-Fluoroorotate was much less toxic to mammalian cells in culture than the commonly used anticancer agent 5-fluorouracil. Unlike malarial parasites in culture, all mammalian cells showed decreased susceptivity to 5-fluoroorotate in the presence of uridine (Table 2; Rathod et al 1989). This was consistent with biochemical observations that mammalian cells, unlike malarial parasites, usually express enzymes for the salvage of pyrimidine nucleosides.

In-vivo Efficacy

Pharmacokinetics of 5-fluoroorotate in mice
In-vitro studies had demonstrated that 0·1–1·0 μM 5-fluoroorotate was sufficient to inhibit proliferation of malarial parasites but not enough to cause significant toxicity to mammalian cells in culture, particularly in the presence of uridine. In an effort to reproduce these conditions in-vivo, mice were injected with varying doses of 5-fluoroorotate and the serum concentrations of 5-fluoroorotate were determined (Gomez & Rathod 1990). Such pharmacokinetic studies revealed that at least 1 mg kg^{-1} of 5-fluoroorotate had to be administered intraperitonneally to obtain 0·1–1·0 μM 5-fluoroorotate in serum. Since the half-life of 5-fluoroorotate was about 90 min, multiple injections of 5-fluoroorotate were anticipated for treating animals infected with malarial parasites.

Curing malaria in mice
Mice harbouring potentially lethal forms of *P. yoelii* at 5% parasitemia could be cured with 5-fluoroorotate without toxicity (Gomez & Rathod 1990; Rathod & Gomez 1991). Doses of 0·2–1·0 mg kg^{-1} six times a day for three days cured all the mice, but only after a significant recrudescence phase. Doses as high as 5 mg kg^{-1} were necessary to avoid recrudescence.

Serum levels necessary to avoid recrudescence
Pharmacokinetics studies had revealed that the doses of 5 mg kg^{-1} in mice produced serum levels of 1–10 μM. These concentrations of 5-fluoroorotate were much higher than those necessary to inhibit the proliferation of *P. falciparum* in culture. If recrudescence was due to resistant parasites, it appeared that 10 μM 5-fluoroorotate may be necessary not just to eliminate the majority of the parasites but to eliminate every single parasite, thereby avoiding resistance.

Uridine rescue to avoid toxicity
Repeated treatment with 5 mg kg^{-1} of 5-fluoroorotate, without uridine, was toxic to mice. In light of the pharmacokinetics, this was not surprising because 10 μM 5-fluoroorotate was toxic to most mammalian cells in the absence of uridine. However, the high doses of 5-fluoroorotate necessary to avoid recrudescence were readily tolerated when uridine was administered with 5-fluoroorotate (Gomez & Rathod 1990; Rathod & Gomez 1991). Mice treated with high doses of 5-fluoroorotate and uridine demonstrated no signs of weight loss, diarrhoea, or leucopenia. Furthermore, while reducing toxicity to the host animal, as seen with malarial parasites in culture, uridine did not compromise the antimalarial potency of 5-fluoroorotate.

Oral availability of 5-fluoroorotate
Mice inoculated with *P. yoelii* were cured by allowing them to drink 5-fluoroorotate freely for three days (Rathod & Gomez 1991). Since mice avoided uridine in the diet or in drinking water, this rescuing nucleoside had to be provided by intraperitoneal injections.

5-Fluoroorotate Resistance

Selection of resistant parasites in-vitro
Malarial parasites exposed to 0·1 μM 5-fluoroorotate generate clones that were 100–400 fold resistant (Rathod et al 1994). Biochemically, the mutant parasites used exogenous orotic acid about 40-fold less efficiently than parental strains. This suggested that the mutants either had diminished capacity to transport exogenous orotate and 5-fluoroorotate or had diminished capacity to activate 5-fluoroorotate to toxic pyrimidine nucleotides. Other explanations seemed less likely. The resistant parasites did not demonstrate increased utilization of exogenous nucleosides. The parasites were not cross-resistant to pyrimethamine, methotrexate, 5-fluorouracil, 5-fluorouridine, or 5-fluoro-2′-deoxyuridine. This suggested that amplification or alteration of dihydrofolate reductase-thymidylate synthase was unlikely to be responsible for 5-fluoroor-

otate resistance The resistance trait was stable in the absence of drug pressure and thus appeared to be of chromosomal origin.

Frequency of 5-fluoroorotate resistance

An in-vitro method was developed to estimate the frequency of resistance of *P. falciparum* to 5-fluoroorotate (Gassis & Rathod 1996). It was demonstrated that *P. falciparum* clone W2, which was already resistant to most antimalarial agents used in the field, developed resistance to $0·1$ μM 5-fluoroorotate with a frequency of 10^{-6}. Recent data from this laboratory indicate that this high frequency may not be common to all clones of malarial parasites (Rathod et al unpublished).

Combinations of 5-fluoroorotate and atovaquone

In addition to 5-fluoroorotate, clone W2 of *P. falciparum* also readily developed resistance to atovaquone (Hudson 1993; Gassis & Rathod 1996). The frequency of resistance to $0·01$ μM atovaquone was 10^{-5}.

Resistance to 5-fluoroorotate and atovaquone could be completely avoided by using a combination of $0·1$ μM 5-fluoroorotate and $0·01$ μM atovaquone (Gassis & Rathod 1996). There was no obvious synergy between 5-fluoroorotate and atovaquone; improved effectiveness was due to lack of cross-resistance between these compounds. Finally, a combination of 5-fluoroorotate and atovaquone did not increase toxicity to mammalian cells. Since these concentrations of antimalarial agents are easily tolerated by mammalian cells in culture, and easily tolerated in serum of mice, it is predicted that a combination of 5-fluoroorotate and atovaquone should eliminate malarial parasites in animals without recrudescence, without toxicity, and without the need to use uridine.

Folate-based Inhibitors of Thymidylate Synthase

New folate-based inhibitors of thymidylate synthase inhibit malarial thymidylate synthase at low nanomolar concentrations (Table 1; Hekmat-Nejad & Rathod 1996). These compounds have enormous potential as new antimalarial agents since their toxicity against mammalian cells, but not malarial cells, can be completely reversed with thymidine (Rathod & Reshmi 1994).

Conclusions

Basic studies on pyrimidine metabolism predicted that 5-fluoroorotate would be a potent and selective inhibitor of malaria proliferation and that this inhibition would be mediated by inactivation of thymidylate synthase. Careful preclinical studies are expected to further pave the way for the use of 5-fluoroorotate in field studies, particularly in combination with other antimalarial agents.

Acknowledgements

P. K. R. is supported by Public Health Service (USA) research grants from the National Institute of Allergy and Infectious Diseases (AI 26912 and AI 01112).

References

Bzik, D. J., Li, W., Horii, T., Insulburg, J. (1987) Molecular cloning and sequence analysis of the *Plasmodium falciparum* dihydrofolate reductase-thymidylate synthetase gene. Proc. Natl Acad. Sci. USA 84: 8360–8364

Carreras, C. W., Santi, D. V. (1995) The catalytic mechanism and structure of thymidylate synthase. Annu. Rev. Biochem. 64: 721–762

Carrington, H. C., Crowther, A. F., Davey, D. G., Levi, A. A., Rose, F. L. (1951) A metabolite of paludrine with high antimalarial activity. Nature 16: 1080

Crabb, B. S., Cowman, A. F. (1996) Characterization of promoters and stable transfection by homologous and non-homologous recombination in *Plasmodium falciparum*. Proc. Natl Acad. Sci. USA 93: 7289–7294

Davisson, V. J., Sirawaraporn, W., Santi, D. V. (1989) Expression of human thymidylate synthase in *Escherichia coli*. J. Biol. Chem. 264: 9145–9148

Dolnick, B. J., Cheng, Y.-C. (1977) Human thymidylate synthetase derived from blast cells of patients with acute myelocytic leukemia. Purification and characterization. J. Biol. Chem. 252: 7697–7703

Donald, R. G. K., Roos, D. S. (1993) Stable molecular transformation of *Toxoplasma gondii*: a selectable dihydrofolate reductase-thymidylate synthase marker based on drug-resistance mutations in malaria. Proc. Natl Acad. Sci. USA 90: 11703–11707

Evans, R. M., Laskin, J. D., Hakala, M. T. (1980) Assessment of growth limiting events caused by 5-fluorouracil in mouse cells and in human cells. Cancer Res. 40: 4113–4122

Ferone, R., Burchall, J. J., Hitchings, G. H. (1969) *Plasmodium bergei* dihydrofolate reductase. Isolation, properties, and inhibition by antifolates. Mol. Pharmacol. 5: 49–59

Foote, S. J., Galatis, D., Cowman, A. F. (1990) Amino acids in the dihydrofolate reductase-thymidylate synthase gene of *Plasmodium falciparum* involved in cycloguanil resistance differ from those involved in pyrimethamine resistance. Proc. Natl Acad. Sci. USA 87: 3014–3017

Garrett, C. E., Coderre, J. A., Meek, T. D., Garvey, E. P., Claman, D., Beverly, S. M., Santi, D. V. (1984) A bifunctional thymidylate synthetase-dihydrofolate reductase in protozoa. Mol. Biochem. Parasitol. 11: 257–265

Gassis, S., Rathod, P. K. (1996) Frequency of drug resistance in *Plasmodium falciparum*: a non-synergistic combination of 5-fluoroorotate and atovaquone suppresses in vitro resistance. Antimicrob. Agents Chemother. 40: 914–919

Gomez, Z., Rathod, P. K. (1990) Antimalarial activity of a 5-fluoroorotate and uridine combination in mice. Antimicrob. Agents Chemother. 34: 1371–1375

Gutteridge, W. E., Trigg, P. I. (1970) Incorporation of radioactive precursors into DNA and RNA of *Plasmodium knowlesi* in vitro. J. Protozool. 17: 89–96

Heidelberger, C., Danenberg, P. V., Moran, R. G. (1983) Fluorinated pyrimidines and their nucleosides. Adv. Enzymol. 54: 57–119

Hekmat-Nejad, M., Rathod, P. K. (1996) Kinetics of *Plasmodium falciparum* thymidylate synthase: interactions with high-affinity metabolites of 5-fluoroorotate and D1694. Antimicrob. Agents Chemother. 40: 1628–1632

Hitchings, G. H. (1960) Pyrimethamine: the use of an antimetabolite in the chemotherapy of malaria and other infections. Clin. Pharmacol. Ther. 1: 570–589

Houghton, P. J., Germain, G. S., Hazelton, B. J., Pennington, J. W., Houghton, J. A. (1989) Mutants of human colon adenocarcinoma, selected for thymidylate synthase deficiency. Proc. Natl Acad. Sci. USA 86: 1377–1381

Hudson, A. T. (1993) Atovaquone – a novel broad-spectrum anti-infective drug. Parasitol. Today 9: 66–68

Ingraham, H. A., Dickey, L., Goulian, M. (1986) DNA fragmentation and cytotoxicity from increased cellular deoxyuridylate. Biochemistry 25: 3225–3230

Jones, M. E. (1980) Pyrimidine biosynthesis of animals: genes, enzymes, and regulation of UMP synthesis. Annu. Rev. Biochem. 49: 253–279

Kunz, B. A., Kohalmi, S. E., Kunkel, T. A., Mathews, C. K., McIntosh, E. M., Reidy, J. A. (1994) Deoxyribonucleoside triphosphate levels: a critical factor in the maintenance of genetic stability. Mutat. Res. 318: 1–64

Moyer, J. D., Malinowski, N., Ayers, O. (1985) Salvage of circulating pyrimidine nucleosides by tissue of the mouse. J. Biol. Chem. 260: 2812–2818

Oaks Jr, S. C., Mitchell, V. S., Pearson, G. W., Pearson, C. C. J. (eds) (1991) Malaria: Obstacles and Opportunities. National Academy Press, Washington, D.C.

Peterson, D. S., Milhous, W. K., Wellems, T. E. (1990) Molecular basis of differential resistance to cycloguanil and pyrimethamine in *Plasmodium falciparum* malaria. Proc. Natl Acad. Sci. USA 87: 3018–3022

Rathod, P. K., Gomez, Z. M. (1991) *Plasmodium yoelii*: oral delivery of 5-fluoroorotate to treat malaria in mice. Exp. Parasitol. 73: 512–514

Rathod, P. K., Reshmi, S. (1994) Susceptibility of *Plasmodium falciparum* to a combination of thymidine and ICI D1694, a quinazoline antifolate directed at thymidylate synthase. Antimicrob. Agents Chemother. 38: 476–480

Rathod, P. K., Reyes, P. (1983) Orotidylate metabolizing enzymes of the human malarial parasite *Plasmodium falciparum*, differ from host cell enzymes. J. Biol. Chem. 258: 2852–2855

Rathod, P. K., Khatri, A., Hubbert, T., Milhous, W. K. (1989) Selective activity of 5-fluoroorotate against *Plasmodium falciparum* in vitro. Antimicrob. Agents Chemother. 33: 1090–1094

Rathod, P. K., Leffers, N. P., Young, R. D. (1992) Molecular targets of 5-fluoroorotate in the human malaria parasite, *Plasmodium falciparum*. Antimicrob. Agents Chemother. 36: 704–711

Rathod, P. K., Khosla, M., Gassis, S., Young, R. D., Lutz, C. (1994) Selection and characterization of 5-fluoroorotate resistant *Plasmodium falciparum*. Antimicrob. Agents Chemother. 38: 2871–2876

Reyes, P., Heidelberger, C. (1965) Fluorinated pyrimidines. XXVI. Mammalian thymidylate synthetase: its mechanism of action and inhibition by fluorinated nucleotides. Mol. Pharmacol. 1: 14–30

Reyes, P., Rathod, P. K., Sanchez, D. J., Mrema, J. E. K., Riekman, K. H., Heidrich, H. G. (1982) Activities of purine and pyrimidine metabolizing enzymes of the human malarial parasite. *Plasmodium falciparum*. Mol. Biochem. Parasitol. 5: 275–290

Santi, D. V. (1981) Inhibition of thymidylate synthase: mechanism, methods, and metabolic consequences. In: Sartorelli, A. C., Lazo, J. S., Bertino, J. R. (eds) Molecular Actions and Targets for Cancer Chemotherapeutic Agents. Academic Press, New York, pp 285–300

Schweitzer, B. I., Dicker, A. P., Bertino, J. R. (1990) Dihydrofolate reductase as a chemotherapeutic target. Fed. Am. Soc. Exp. Biol. J. 4: 2441–2452

Sherman, I. W. (1979) Biochemistry of *Plasmodium* (malarial parasites). Microbiol. Rev. 43: 453–495

Sirawaraporn, W., Sirawaraporn, R., Cowman, A. F., Yuthavong, Y., Santi, D. V. (1990) Heterologous expression of active thymidylate synthase-dihydrofolate reductase from *Plasmodium falciparum*. Biochemistry 29: 10779–10785

van Dijk, M. R., Janse, C. J., Waters, A. P. (1996) Expression of a *Plasmodium* gene introduced into subtelomeric regions of *Plasmodium berghei* chromosomes. Science 271: 662–665

Wu, Y., Kirkman, L. A., Wellems, T. E. (1996) Transformation of *Plasmodium falciparum* malaria parasites by homologous integration of plasmids that confer resistance to pyrimethamine. Proc. Natl Acad. Sci. USA 93: 1130–1134

White, N. J. (1996) The treatment of malaria. N. Engl. J. Med. 335: 800–806

Yoshioka, A., Tanaka, S., Hiraoka, O., Koyama, Y., Hirota, Y., Ayusawa, D., Seno, T., Garrett, C., Wataya, Y. (1987) Deoxyribonucleoside triphosphate imbalance. 5-Fluorodeoxyuridine-induced DNA double strand breaks in mouse FM3A cells and the mechanism of cell death. J. Biol. Chem. 262: 8235–8241

Young, R. D., Rathod, P. K. (1993) Clonal viability measurements on *Plasmodium falciparum* to assess in vitro schizonticidal activity of leupeptin, chloroquine, and 5-fluoroorotate. Antimicrob. Agents Chemother. 37: 1102–1107

Zolg, J. W., Plitt, J. R., Chen, G.-X., Palmer, S. (1989) Point mutations in the dihydrofolate reductase-thymidylate synthase gene as the molecular basis for pyrimethamine resistance in *Plasmodium falciparum*. Mol. Biochem. Parasitol. 36: 253–262

J. Pharm. Pharmacol. 1997, 49 (Suppl. 2): 71–76

The DNA Replisome of the Malaria Parasite: Progress Towards a Useful Drug Target

BRIAN J. KILBEY

Institute of Cell and Molecular Biology, University of Edinburgh, Edinburgh EH9 3JR, UK

The enzymes and auxilliary proteins that cooperate to bring about the replication of the eukaryotic genome have the potential to be a set of very important drug targets. DNA is replicated every time a cell divides and, in the case of Plasmodium, there are five distinct points in its life cycle when this occurs (White & Kilbey 1996). The selective blocking of DNA synthesis in the parasite should inhibit both the disease itself and its transmission. In this presentation the essential features of eukaryotic DNA replication will be outlined briefly and then the attempts we are making to develop the replication system of the parasite as a source of new drug targets will be described. This should be regarded as a progress report—the task is far from complete.

Eukaryotic DNA Replication

Most of the basic information concerning the DNA replication proteins and their function has been derived from experiments in which an in vitro synthesizing system has been reconstructed with proteins purified from animal cells. The templates in these experiments are either the Simian virus (SV40) genome itself or plasmids which have an SV40 origin of replication. The system is believed to be a good model for chromosomal replication because the only non-host cell protein needed is the large viral T antigen (Stillman 1994; Waga & Stillman 1994).

Chromosomal DNA replication proceeds in two phases: firstly, an initiation phase during which short RNA primers are synthesized at the replication origin and DNA synthesis is initiated by DNA polymerase α (DNAPolα); and secondly, an elongation phase in which the relatively error-prone and less processive DNAPolα is replaced by the highly processive and accurate combination of DNAPolδ and proliferating cell nuclear antigen (PCNA). PCNA is a homotrimer which appears to act as a clamp maintaining contact between the DNA polymerase and its template. Other proteins are also involved. There is a group of origin recognition proteins whose function appears to be to assemble the replicative machinery at the replication origin and to activate it. Strand unwinding at the origin and thereafter is facilitated by the action of topoisomerases I/II. The single strands of DNA produced by unwinding the duplex are protected by their association with a heterotrimeric complex (RF-A) which may also have a role to play in the overall regulation of DNA replication (Din et al 1990). The switch from DNAPolα to DNAPolδ requires the participation of a further complex of five polypeptides, RF-C. This group of proteins recognizes the 3'OH end of the nascent strand and recruits PCNA and DNAPolδ in an ATP-dependent manner displacing DNAPolα from the template. A 50-kDa subunit is always found associated with DNAPolδ and, although its precise role has not been ascertained, its ubiquity

and conservation suggests it has an important part to play in the synthetic process. Other proteins of importance include enzymes which remove RNA primers and ligate together Okazaki fragments. A third DNA polymerase, DNAPolε may also play an essential part although its precise role remains unclear. All in all, then, we are considering a process which requires the cooperation of about 20 proteins for its execution. The essential nature of the individual components has been clearly demonstrated by studying the cell cycle arrest phenotypes of temperature sensitive mutations which affect the function of these homologues in yeast. When cells harbouring any one of these mutations are incubated at the restrictive temperature, progression through the cell cycle is arrested at the onset of S phase showing that loss of the function prevents the completion of DNA synthesis.

Antimalarials and DNA Replication

Some antimalarial drugs interfere with DNA synthesis indirectly by restricting the supply of DNA precursors (e.g. the folic acid antagonist, pyrimethamine). However, this discussion focusses on two groups of compounds which may target the DNA replication mechanism more directly. These are the acyclic nucleosides as exemplified by HPMPA (*S*-9-(3-hydroxy-2-phosphonylmethoxypropyl)adenine) and the 9-anilino acridines (Fig. 1).

HPMPA was chosen as a possible inhibitor of DNA replication on the basis of its action in viral systems (de Vries et al 1991). *Plasmodium falciparum* growing in culture was shown to be inhibited by HPMPA in a concentration-dependent manner. At 4×10^{-7} M, HPMPA completely blocked parasite growth and it was estimated that the parasite is approximately 1500 times more sensitive to the compound than the human

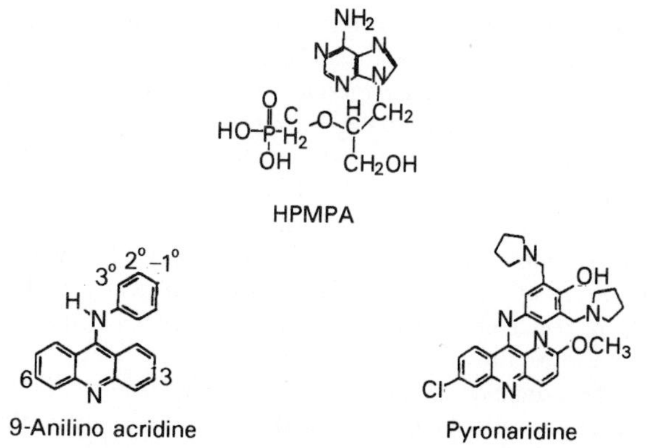

FIG. 1. Chemical structures of antimalarial compounds referred to in text.

embryonic lung cells used for comparison. The effects of the analogue were not reversed by washing. A 3-deaza derivative of HPMPA appeared to be even more effective. The ID50 determined 72 h after the drug was administered to the cultured cells was 47 nM for HPMPA but only 8 nM for the 3-deaza derivative. Intraperitoneal administration of a single dose of HPMPA (20 mg kg^{-1}) to mice infected with *P. berghei* at a parasitaemia of 3·5–4% prevented any further increase in parasitaemia for four days, but after four days it increased to control levels. Repeated dosing reduced parasitaemia to barely detectable levels but again, once dosing was stopped, parasitaemia increased.

Since these agents were believed to act directly on the DNA polymerizing system, attempts were made to identify the fraction of polymerase activity being targeted. Identification of specific polymerase activities in the malaria parasite is extremely difficult, but it was possible to show that HeLa DNA polymerase α and aphidicolin-sensitive fractions (believed to be equivalent to α) in both *P. falciparum* and *P. berghei* were equally sensitive (IC50 of ~40 μM) to the phosphorylated metabolic derivative of HPMPA, HPMPApp. Perhaps surprisingly, the most sensitive polymerase was the aphidicolin-resistant fraction (possibly corresponding to a mitochondrial γ-like polymerase) from *P. falciparum* (IC50 = 1 μM) although the same activity fraction from *P. berghei* was rather resistant with an IC50 over 500 times greater. Lineweaver–Burke plots using the aphidicolin-sensitive fraction from *P. berghei* suggested that the acyclic nucleoside could compete with dATP for the enzyme in-vitro. A subsequent examination of the kinetics of inhibition of DNA synthesis in intact *P. falciparum* has, however, cast doubt on the primary action of these inhibitors (Smeijsters et al 1994). When inhibitory doses of the analogue were used to treat parasites embarking on schizogony, it quickly became clear that the synthesis of chromosomal DNA did not stop immediately but continued until 8 times the haploid DNA level was reached. Furthermore, the synthesis of mitochondrial and plastid-like DNA was not inhibited although, as noted above, the most sensitive polymerase fraction appeared to be that most readily associated with mitochondrial DNA replication. In other words, the data suggest that the DNA polymerases may not be the most important targets of the drug in the intact parasite and other explanations of the observations are needed. A suggestion that the unfavourable K_i/K_m values might imply the depletion of intracellular dATP levels with the consequent slowing of DNA synthesis was readily discounted. Similarly, inhibition of ribonucleotide reductase and depression in the supply of DNA precursor molecules could also be discounted on the basis of direct tests. Incorporation of the analogue leading to progressive chain termination or mutation accumulation was also eliminated as a possibility. The issue thus remains unresolved. One possibility which has not so far been considered is that, instead of a precursor molecule being depleted, one or more of the replisome components may cease to be made under the influence of the analogue and become sufficiently depleted during the course of nuclear division to cause the synthesis of DNA to be arrested.

The 9-anilino acridines provide a second example, in particular, the related compound pyronaridine (Fig. 1). 9-Anilino acridines are active as topoisomerase II poisons and their 3,6-diamino derivatives appear to be selectively effective in the inhibition of parasite metabolism as measured by the incorporation of ^{3}[H]hypoxanthine (Chavalitshewinkoon et al 1993; Gamage et al 1994). Direct evidence that they inhibit topoisomerase II activity in the parasite was obtained from experiments in which they were shown to inhibit DNA decatenation by parasite extracts. The causal connection between these two activities has, however, still to be established. Pyronaridine itself was developed in China about ten years ago (Fu & Xiao 1991) and has proved effective in clinical trials against chloroquine-resistant parasites. In-vitro tests suggest that mammalian cells, in this case Jurkat leukaemia cells, are 500 to 1000 times more resistant to the chemical than the parasite but this is a relatively crude index. These results are very tantalizing and what we really need is more information on the precise mode of action of pyronaridine. Is its sole target topoisomerase II, or are other targets more important for its antimalarial action? Are there any drugs which incapacitate the parasite simply by inactivating its topoisomerase activity? An understanding of the basis of resistance to the action of these agents would help to answer these questions and also, in particular, evidence that parasites resistant to pyronaridine, for example, have mutationally altered topoisomerase II.

Some of these questions illustrate the sort of problems often encountered in trying to determine the mode of action of an antimalarial drug and the importance of adopting molecular strategies for the study of parasite replication proteins. For this reason, apart from the practical difficulties of producing enough parasite material for standard biochemical study, we have been isolating and studying the DNA sequences which encode the essential replication proteins of *P. falciparum*. Our objective is to over-express them heterologously and build up an in vitro system for DNA replication which will be useful both for studying its basic characteristics and its selective inhibition by potential antimalarial agents. We are also interested in determining the mechanisms which control the synthesis of these proteins since these may provide us with additional opportunities for therapeutic action. The rest of this presentation describes the progress we have made towards realizing these objectives.

Genes Encoding Parasite Replication Proteins

Our primary approach to the isolation of the genes encoding the parasite's replication proteins has been to design degenerate oligonucleotide probes based upon evolutionarily conserved regions of the proteins and to use them for screening genomic and cDNA parasite libraries. Latterly we have used the polymerase chain reaction to amplify a fragment of the gene in question for use as a library probe and we have also used heterologous probes derived from yeast. We are currently considering the use of protein–protein interactions as a way of augmenting the probing approach which relies heavily on the availability of comparative sequence data. Since we commenced this work in 1990 we have identified the sequences of nine of the genes which encode the parasite's DNA replication proteins. Five of these are fully characterised and the others will soon be completed. The structures of the proteins predicted by the first five genes we studied are presented in Fig. 2. In addition to the genes we are working with, the gene encoding the small subunit of DNA primase has also been isolated and characterized (de Vries, personal communication).

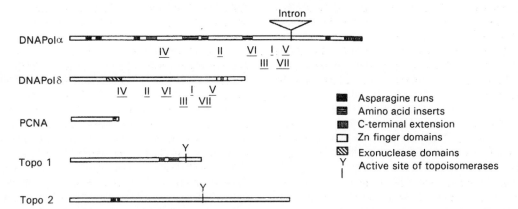

FIG. 2. The maps of the predicted protein products encoded by DNA replication genes of the human malarial parasite strain K1. The data were derived from the following sources: DNA polymerase α (White et al 1993); DNA polymerase δ (Ridley et al 1992); PCNA (Kilbey et al 1993); topoisomerase I (Tosh & Kilbey 1995); topoisomerase II (Cheesman et al 1994).

Eukaryotic replicative DNA polymerases are characterized by seven conserved motifs. The DNA polymerases of *P. falciparum* are no exception and the motifs are present in the same order as in other polymerases (labelled I-VII in Fig. 2). In addition, PfDNAPolα has some of the features which are characteristic of α-type DNA polymerases. There are usually five of these which are referred to as A-E (White & Kilbey 1996). The functions associated with many of these conserved sequences are not known although the highly conserved motif I probably contributes to the active site of the polymerase and some others may represent substrate binding sites. Motif A is absent from the *P. falciparum* sequence and there is a unique substitution of glycine by leucine in the D motif of *P. falciparum*. This residue has been implicated in the reaction between polymerase and primase in yeast (Luccini et al 1988, 1990). PfDNAPolδ is the least divergent of the replication proteins and possesses all the features which characterize a DNA polymerase and, in addition, the amino terminal exonuclease domains which are implicated in the editing activity of the enzyme as described for *Saccharomyces cerevisiae* (Simon et al 1991). It also possesses two putative Zinc finger domains towards the carboxy terminus which are of unknown significance. PfPCNA, the processivity factor for PfDNAPolδ is the smallest of these proteins. The sequence matches rather closely the sequences of human and yeast PCNAs and, in collaboration with Shane Sturrock of The Institute of Cell and Molecular Biology, University of Edinburgh, we have produced a structure for PfPCNA using the coordinates derived from X-ray diffraction data from the yeast homologue. When these predicted proteins are compared with their homologues from other species it is immediately apparent that many of them have extra tracts of amino acids in their sequence. The only exception so far has been PfDNAPolδ. Since these are only predicted amino acid sequences, we cannot be certain that the additional blocks of amino acid residues will be found when the native proteins are purified and sequenced. All we can say at present is that comparisons between cDNA and genomic DNA sequences show that the nucleotides which encode them are not removed from the gene transcripts when the latter are processed and we must therefore assume they are part of the final translated product. These additional tracts are sometimes asparagine-rich and two of them in PfDNAPolα

include several copies of six-amino-acid motifs of the type often reported for parasite antigens. The function of the repeated motifs is unknown and, indeed, they may have no function. There is evidence that the repeat number in PfDNAPolα may vary from isolate to isolate (de Vries, cited in White & Kilbey 1996). Because of these inserted sequences, the overall percentage similarity between these proteins and their homologues in other species can often be quite low. In the case of PfDNAPolα, for example, the figure is below 20%. Within the functional core of the enzyme the figure is higher. Unfortunately these figures are not a reliable guide to the utility of these proteins as selective drug targets.

Each of the genes we have isolated and studied represents a unique coding sequence in the genome and each has been mapped to a specific chromosome, although not to a chromosomal region as yet.

Heterologous Expression

The ultimate aim of the work we are doing is to over-express the full length recombinant proteins in a convenient heterologous system and to purify them in an active form. There is no a priori way of identifying a suitable system for expression and we have tried using baculovirus-infected Sf9 cells, fungi and *Escherichia coli* for this purpose with varying degrees of success. John White and Jennifer Daub have had some success with expressing both PfDNAPolδ and PfPCNA in *E. coli* and PfPCNA in the baculovirus system. Sandie Cheesman has successfully expressed topoisomerase II in the baculovirus system. Their results will be reported in detail elsewhere and I shall discuss them only briefly here, concentrating on PfPCNA.

PfPCNA is a protein of 30.5 kDa encoded by a sequence of 825nt. The sequence has no introns but, as noted earlier, it does include a nine-amino-acid insertion near the carboxy terminus. The full length, soluble protein has been expressed either fused in frame with glutathione-*S*-transferase (GST) in *E. coli* or with a polyhistidine tag in insect cells. The tags facilitate one step purification of the recombinant protein using affinity columns. The affinity tags have been successfully removed with the appropriate protease yielding soluble full length protein. The conditions of expression are important. When PfPCNA is expressed as a histidine-tagged product from a polH promoter in insect cells, the best results (high yield with no degradation) are obtained when harvesting is done 24 h after infection of the host cells with the expression construct. Although more material is obtained at longer times, degradation increases the problems of purification. An antiserum raised against a PfPCNA fragment (Kilbey et al 1993) recognizes the affinity-tagged recombinant material as well as the full-length material and the endogenous protein. Similar results have been obtained using a GST fusion with *E. coli*. Highly purified recombinant PfPCNA is now available and light-scattering experiments strongly suggest that it trimerizes spontaneously presumably adopting its functional, toroidal conformation. We hope to be able to use this material for crystallization to confirm the structure predicted on the basis of the coordinates published for the yeast homologue. The results with PfDNAPolδ have also been encouraging. Although all attempts to produce an immunologically identifiable, histidine-tagged protein in insect cells have failed, full-length GST-tagged protein has been generated in *E. coli*. Currently the material is not completely purified, but an attempt is being made to set up a basic in vitro replication system based on recombinant PfDNAPolδ and PfPCNA. At this point we do not know whether additional polypeptides are necessary to facilitate the PfDNAPolδ/PfPCNA interaction. One of these may be a 50-kDa subunit which is found associated with the polymerase when it is purified from mammalian cell extracts. We have isolated the structural gene for its parasite homologue (Wilson & Kilbey, unpublished data).

Regulation of DNA Replication Gene Activity

The mutational studies with yeast which demonstrated the essential nature of the individual components of the DNA replisome have shown that the absence of just one active component can stall synthesis indefinitely. We have therefore become interested in the mechanisms which regulate the expression of the genes encoding the parasite's replication proteins, since an ability to manipulate their expression might provide a highly effective and selective way of controlling parasite growth. The parasite synthesizes its DNA at five discrete points in its complex life cycle (White & Kilbey 1996). Two of these episodes take place in the human host during the parasites' development in the liver and in the erythrocytes. The remainder take place in the mosquito during male gametogenesis, just prior to meiosis shortly after fertilization and, finally, during the formation of hundreds of sporozoites. There may be other points at which the cellular DNA increases but these are less well understood and may not represent duplication of the whole genome. The control networks which activate the programme of DNA replication are not understood but they presumably involve surface receptors and signal transduction pathways. However, whatever the details may be, adequate supplies of the catalytic enzymes and cofactors needed for DNA replication must be synthesised to carry through often several rounds of genome replication. The regulation of the genes encoding these proteins in the parasite has not been studied hitherto but we have now embarked on a study of the regulation of the genes at our disposal starting with the two key components of the system, PfPCNA and PfDNAPolδ. Our work so far has been limited to studying the expression of these two genes during the intraerythrocytic

stages since these are readily cultured in human blood and the growing parasites can be readily synchronized (Lambros & Vanderberg 1979). RNA and proteins have been extracted from synchronized populations of parasites and, by means of northern and western analysis, we have followed the appearance of PfPCNA and PfDNAPolδ and their messages as the parasites prepare to synthesize DNA. At the same time nuclear extracts have been prepared and nuclear run-on experiments conducted to provide information on stage-specific promoter activity (Horrocks et al 1996). DNA synthesis is known to take place during schizogony and we had already shown by means of immunofluorescence analysis that the levels of PfPCNA increase rapidly in late trophozoites, and remain high in schizonts (Kilbey et al 1993). Western analysis confirmed this pattern and showed that, on a per-cell basis, the levels of PfPCNA and PfDNAPolδ behaved similarly. Northern analysis provided little or no evidence of the messages for these proteins in ring stage parasites but abundant messages were found in the trophozoite samples, although there was a substantial decrease in schizonts. Synchronization is never complete but, by using diagnostic probes to genes with known patterns of expression we were able to confirm the reality of our observations. In contrast to the pattern of accumulation of messages and proteins, we found that promoter activity differed between the two genes. Although the PfDNAPolδ promoter activity paralleled the levels of message and protein at the different stages of intraerythrocytic development, PfPCNA promoter activity was found at all stages of intraerythrocytic parasite development, including rings. These data suggest that, although the products of the two genes appear simultaneously, they are probably under different mechanisms of control. Until recently this is as far as studies of gene regulation in the parasite could go. Although several 5′ flanking regions have been studied intensively and potential regulatory elements identified, it has been impossible to test the validity of the proposals because transfection with mutationally modified promoters has been impossible. This has changed with the very recent discovery that it is possible to introduce exogenous DNA into asexual parasites by electroporation. The first successful experiments were actually done with gametes and fertilized zygotes of *P. gallanaceum* since these are readily available and are free-living parasites (Goonewardene et al 1993) but, since then, electroporation has been used successfully with the blood stages of both human (Wu et al 1995) and rodent (van Dijk et al 1996) malarias. We have started our investigation by studying the effects of various mutations on PfPCNA promoter activity as measured by the expression of the reporter gene, firefly luciferase (*luc*). Experiments done in Tom Wellems' laboratory at NIH showed that this gene is expressed in the parasite when placed under the control of the HRP3 promoter (Wu et al 1995) and we were able to show that the 5′ flanking region of PfPCNA could also drive *luc* gene expression in the parasite (Horrocks & Kilbey 1996). The 5′ PfPCNA sequence was then modified by manipulating the restriction fragments and by using the polymerase chain reaction to generate specific deletions and a segmental inversion before fusing the modified sequences to the *luc* reporter gene. Each construct in turn was electroporated into ring stage parasites and the parasites cultured for 48 h before harvesting. A sample was scored for parasitaemia but the remaining material was extracted and assayed for luciferase activity using

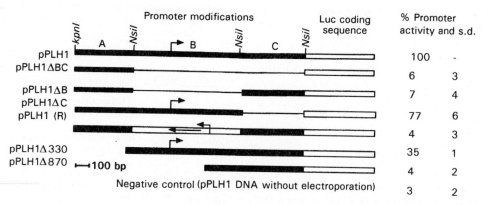

FIG. 3. Relative promoter activity of a series of mutationally modified PfPCNA promoters. Internal deletions are indicated by single lines. The major transcriptional start site is indicated and the reverse orientations of segment B in pPLH (R). Activities are expressed as percentages of the promoter activity of the full-length construct. s.d. = standard deviation. Each construct was tested at least twice. Data extracted from Horrocks & Kilbey (1996).

an Argus photon camera and image processor. A summary of the data is provided in Fig. 3. If the central region is deleted or inverted, expression is abolished. This is consistent with our mapping of the putative transcriptional start sites to this region. Furthermore, even if only the part of this central region containing the putative transcriptional start sites is deleted, activity is also lost. There is also evidence that other elements may be important for expression. Removal of the distal 400 nucleotides of upstream sequence reduces the promoter activity to about a third of the maximal rate. Presumably this region contains elements which enhance promoter activity although we still have to verify the enhancer status of the segment and identify the elements involved. The proximal 400 nucleotides appear to be much less significant since their removal only reduces activity by about 25%. We hope to be able to pinpoint the regulatory elements precisely by the use of a more extensive deletion analysis and with directed mutation and we shall try to identify the regulatory factors which recognize them and to isolate the genes which encode them. This has clear scientific interest in its own right but we also hope that it will eventually extend our scope for intervention in the control of this disease.

Conclusions

The control of malaria is a pressing problem which we can only hope to attack by extending our understanding of the parasite's cell biology. DNA synthesis represents one cellular system which is amenable to study and it may also provide a source of targets which will be most useful in attacking the organism selectively. We are now within sight of isolating the parasite homologues of all the genes known to play a part in DNA synthesis and we have started to examine the controls which regulate their activity. We have also shown that it is possible to express some of these genes in heterologous systems and we hope soon to have an in-vitro system which will be useful as a tool for evaluating the antimalarial action of DNA replication inhibitors and in understanding their function.

Acknowledgements

This work owes everything to the commitment and perseverence of my colleagues, John White, Sandie Cheesman, Kerrie Tosh, Paul Horrocks, Jennifer Daub and Jill Douglas. I am glad to acknowledge their collaboration, and that of earlier co-workers, in particular of Robert Ridley. I am also grateful for discussions with Richard Carter and Ali Aloueche. The work is funded by the Medical Research Council.

References

Chavalitshewinkoon, P., Wiliarat, P., Gamage, S., Denny,W., Figgitt, D., Ralph, R. (1993) Structure-activity relationships and modes of action of 9-anilino acridines against chloroquine-resistant *Plasmodium falciparum*. Antimicrob. Agents Chemother. 37: 403–406

Cheesman, S., McAleese, S., Goman, M., Johnson, D., Horrocks, P., Ridley, R. G., Kilbey, B. J.(1994) The gene encoding topoisomerase II from *Plasmodium falciparum*. Nucleic Acids Res. 22: 2547–2551

de Vries, E., Stam, J. G., Franssen, F. F. J., Nieuwenhuijs, H., Chavalitshewinkoon, P., de Clercq, E., Overdulve, J. P., van der Vliet, P. (1991) Inhibition of the growth of *Plasmodium falciparum* and *Plasmodium berghei* by the DNA polymerase inhibitor HPMPA. Mol. Biochem. Parasitol. 47: 43–50

Din, S., Brill, S. J., Fairman, M. P., Stillman, B. (1990) Cell-cycle-regulated phosphorylation of DNA replication factor A from human and yeast cells. Genes Dev. 4: 968–977

Fu, S., Xiao, S-H. (1991) Pyronaridine: a new antimalarial drug. Parasitol. Today 7: 310–313

Gamage, S. A., Tepsiri, N., Wiliarat, P., Wojcik,S. J., Figgitt, D., Ralph, R., Denny,W. (1994) Synthesis and in vitro evaluation of 9-aniline 3-6-diaminoacridines active against a multidrug resistant strain of the malaria parasite. J. Med. Chem. 37: 1486–1494

Goonewardene, R., Daily, J., Kaslow, D., Sullivan, T. J., Duffy, P., Carter, R., Mendis, K., Wirth, D. (1993) Transfection of the malaria parasite and expression of firefly luciferase. Proc. Natl Acad. Sci. USA 90: 5234–5236

Horrocks, P., Kilbey, B. J. (1996) Physical and functional mapping of the transcriptional start sites of *Plasmodium falciparum* proliferating cell nuclear antigen. Mol. Biochem. Parasitol. 82: 207–215

Horrocks, P., Jackson, M., Cheesman, S., White, J. H., Kilbey, B. J. (1996) Stage specific expression of proliferating cell nuclear antigen and DNA polymerase δ from *Plasmodium falciparum*. Mol. Biochem. Parasitol. 79: 177–182

Kilbey, B. J., Fraser, I., McAleese, S., Goman, M., Ridley, R. G. (1993) Molecular characterisation and the stage specific expression of proliferating cell nuclear antigen (PCNA) from the malarial parasite *Plasmodium falciparum*. Nucleic Acids Res. 21: 239–243

Lambros, C., Vanderberg, S. P. (1979) Synchronisation of *Plasmodium falciparum* erythrocytic stages in cultures. J. Parasitol. 65: 418–420

Luccini, G., Mazza, C., Scacheri, E., Plevani, P. (1988) Genetic mapping of the *Saccharomyces cerevisiae* DNA polymerase 1 gene and characterisation of a Pol1 temperature-sensitive mutant altered in DNA primase-polymerase complex stability. Mol. Gen. Genet. 212: 459–465

Luccini, G., Falconi, M. M., Pizzagalli, A., Aguilera, A., Klein, H. L., Plevani, P. (1990) Nucleotide sequence and characterisation of temperature-sensitive pol1 mutants of *Saccharomyces cerevisiae*. Gene 90: 99–104

Ridley, R. G., White, J. M., McAlease, S. M., Gorman, M., Alaine, P., de Vries, E., Kilbey, B. J. (1991) DNA polymeraseδ gene sequences from *Plasmodium falciparum* indicate that the enzyme is more highly conserved than DNA plymerase α. Nucleic acids Res. 19: 6731–6736

Simon, M., Giot, L., Faye, G. (1991) The 3′ to 5′ exonuclease activity located in the DNA polymerase δ subunit of *Saccharomyces cerevisiae* is required for accurate replication. EMBO J. 10: 2165–2170

Stillman, B. (1994) Smart machines at the DNA replication fork. Cell 78: 725–728

Smeijsters, L. J. J. W., Zijlstra, N. M., de Vries, E., Franssen, F. F. J., Janse, C. J., Overdulve, J. P. (1994) The effect of (*S*)-9-(3-hydroxy-2-phosphonylmethoxypropyl)adenine on nuclear and organellar DNA synthesis in erythrocytic schizogony in malaria. Mol. Biochem. Parasitol. 67: 115–124

Tosh, K., Kilbey, B. J. (1995) The gene encoding topoisomerase I from the human malaria parasite, *Plasmodium falciparum*. Gene 163: 151–154

van Dijk, M. R., Janse, C. J., Waters, A. P. (1996) Stable transfection of malaria parasite blood stages. Science 271: 662–665

Waga, S., Stillman, B. (1994) Anatomy of a DNA replication fork revealed by reconstitution of SV40 DNA replication in vitro. Nature 369: 207–212

White, J. H., Kilbey, B. J. (1996) DNA replication in the malaria parasite. Parasitol. Today 12: 151–155

White, J. H., Kilbey, B. J., de Vries, E., Goman, M., Alano, P., Cheesman, S., McAleese, S., Ridley, R. G. (1993) The gene encoding DNA polymerase α from *Plasmodium falciparum*. Nucleic Acids Res. 21: 3643–3646

Wu, Y., Sifri, C. D., Lei, H-H., Su, X-H., Wellems, T. E. (1995) Transfection of *Plasmodium falciparum* within human red blood cells. Proc. Natl Acad. Sci. USA 92: 973–977

Journal of

Pharmacy and Pharmacology

VOLUME 49 • SUPPLEMENT 2 • APRIL 1997

SUBJECT INDEX

Journal of
Pharmacy and Pharmacology

VOLUME 49 • SUPPLEMENT 2 • APRIL 1997

AUTHOR INDEX

New Books from the Pharmaceutical Press

MARTINDALE

The Extra Pharmacopoeia

Thirty-First Edition

The renowned, authoritative source of evaluated information on the world's drugs and medicines

Prepared by editorial staff of the Royal Pharmaceutical Society of Great Britain and edited by Dr James E. F. Reynolds

This new edition of Martindale is more up-to-date, contains more material and is simpler to use than any previous edition. The epitome of clarity, it provides succinct and authoritative information on drugs and medicines that are used throughout the world. It is an invaluable resource for health professionals.

'an essential reference for pharmacists in all branches of the profession.'

The Pharmaceutical Journal, 1993;250: 582

The 31st edition is:

- **Forty percent larger containing more critical reviews, more preparations from a wider coverage of countries**

- **More up-to-date, all chapters completely revised and updated**

- **Simpler to use**

  - **Stronger, clearer links between preparations and monographs**

  - **Improved, redesigned layout**

  - **Increased clinical emphasis giving greater perspective to the different treatments**

Publication date: April 1996   Price: £176   Overseas Price: £187   Members Price: £160
Extent: 2800pp   ISBN: 0 85369 342 0

ORDER FORM

To: The Pharmaceutical Press, PO Box 151, Wallingford, Oxon OX10 8QU, Telephone (01491) 824 486, Fax (01491) 826 090, E-Mail: rpsgb@cabi.org

Please supply _____ copy/copies of Martindale: The Extra Pharmacopoeia published by The Pharmaceutical Press at the special members price of £160 per copy.

Please supply _____ copy/copies of Martindale: The Extra Pharmacopoeia published by The Pharmaceutical Press at £176.00 per copy. Overseas Price: £187 per copy.

My cheque/money order for £ _____ is enclosed.

My credit card number is_____
Visa / Access / Eurocard / Mastercard

Expiry date _____ Date _____

Signature _____
Name: _____
Full postal address: _____
_____
_____

Companies in EC member states (excluding the UK) must supply VAT identifying number (TVA/BTW/MOMS/MWST/IVA/FPA)

_____

If the address for your credit card account is not the same as that above, please give this separately.
☐ Please do not add my name to your mailing list